STUDENT WORKBOOK AND RESOURCE GUIDE FOR

PHARMACOLOGY FOR NURSES

A Pathophysiologic Approach

FOURTH EDITION

MICHAEL PATRICK ADAMS, PhD

Professor of Anatomy and Physiology
St. Petersburg College
Formerly Dean of Health Professions
Pasco-Hernando Community College

LELAND NORMAN HOLLAND, Jr., PhD

Program Manager
Hillsborough Community College
SouthShore Campus and
Professor of Pharmacology,
MSN Nursing Program
Liberty University

PEARSON

Boston   Columbus   Indianapolis   New York   San Francisco   Upper Saddle River
Amsterdam   Cape Town   Dubai   London   Madrid   Milan   Munich   Paris   Montreal   Toronto
Delhi   Mexico City   Sao Paulo   Sydney   Hong Kong   Seoul   Singapore   Taipei   Tokyo

Publisher: Julie Levin Alexander
Assistant to Publisher: Regina Bruno
Executive Acquisitions Editor: Pamela Fuller
Development Editor: Anne Seitz, Hearthside Publishing Services
Assistant Editor: Cynthia Gates
Director of Marketing: David Gesell
Marketing Coordinator: Michael Sirinides
Managing Editor, Production: Patrick Walsh
Production Editor: Shyam Ramasubramony, S4Carlisle Publishing Services
Production Liaison: Cathy O'Connell
Media Project Manager: Leslie Brado
Manufacturing Manager: Lisa McDowell
Art Director: Christopher Weigand
Composition: S4Carlisle Publishing Services
Printer/Binder: Edwards Brothers Malloy
Cover Printer: Edwards Brothers Malloy
Cover Printer: Lehigh/Phoenix Color Hagerstown

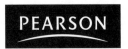

www.pearsonhighered.com

10 9 8 7 6 5 4 3 2 1
ISBN 13: 978-0-13-338972-2
ISBN 10: 0-13-338972-3

CONTENTS

PREFACE

Students entering the field of nursing have a tremendous amount to learn in a very short time. This concise student workbook and resource guide has been developed to help you learn and apply key concepts and procedures, and master critical-thinking skills based on *Pharmacology for Nurses: A Pathophysiologic Approach,* Fourth Edition.

Each chapter includes a variety of questions and activities to help you comprehend difficult concepts and reinforce basic knowledge gained from textbook reading assignments. Highlights of this workbook include:

- Chapters that correlate directly to *Pharmacology for Nurses: A Pathophysiologic Approach,* Fourth Edition to allow you to easily locate information related to each question.
- Thorough assessment of essential information in the chapter through generous use of multiple-choice, fill-in-the-blank, and matching style questions.
- Making Connections questions encourage you to recall concepts from previous chapters and apply them to the current chapter, thus promoting retention of information and continuity of learning.
- Dosage calculation problems provide additional practice to assist you in mastering this challenging topic.
- Case study applications provide in-depth scenarios to sharpen critical-thinking skills.
- Answers are included in an appendix to provide immediate reinforcement and to allow you to check the accuracy of your work.

It is our hope that this workbook contributes to your success in beginning the study of the exciting and challenging subject of pharmacology.

Pearson Nursing Student Resources
Find additional review materials at nursing.pearsonhighered.com.
Prepare for success with additional NCLEX®-style practice questions,
interactive assignments and activities, Web links, animations and
videos, and more!

CHAPTER 1

INTRODUCTION TO PHARMACOLOGY

FILL IN THE BLANK

From the textbook, find the correct word(s) to complete the statement(s).

1. _____ is the father of American pharmacology.

2. In the early days of pharmacology, _____ had to isolate active agents from scarce _____ to create drugs used to treat patients.

3. In the 20th century, chemists and pharmacologists learned to _____ their own drugs in the laboratory.

4. The central purpose of pharmacology focuses on improving the _____.

5. Pharmacology is defined as the study of _____.

6. Therapeutics is the branch of medicine concerned with the prevention of _____.

7. Pharmacotherapeutics is the application of drugs for the purpose of disease _____ and treatment of _____.

8. A drug is a chemical agent capable of producing _____ responses within the body.

9. _____ drugs do not require a physician's order.

Adams/Holland, *Student Workbook and Resource Guide for Pharmacology for Nurses* 4th Edition
© 2014 by Pearson Education, Inc.

MATCHING

For questions 10 through 13, match the concept in column I with the agent in column II.

Column I	Column II
10. _____ biologics	a. morphine
11. _____ alternative therapies	b. hormones
12. _____ active agent	c. herbs
13. _____ nontherapeutic	d. sunscreen

For questions 14 through 17, match the concept in column I with the definition in column II.

Column I	Column II
14. _____ formulary	a. standards for drugs
15. _____ pharmacopeia	b. list of drugs
16. _____ USP label	c. drug regulation
17. _____ Biologics Control Act	d. exact amount of ingredient

MULTIPLE CHOICE

18. The Pure Food and Drug Act of 1906 gave the government power to do what?

    a. Sell OTC products

    b. Synthesize morphine

    c. Control drug labeling

    d. Open pharmacy companies

19. The Food, Drug, and Cosmetic Act of 1938 prevented which of the following?

    a. Use of herbal products

    b. Synthesis of narcotic substances

    c. Distribution of dietary supplements

    d. Sale of drugs that had not been thoroughly tested

20. The FDA is NOT responsible for overseeing the administration of which of the following products?

    a. Dietary supplements

    b. Herbal products

    c. OTC drugs

    d. Pesticides

21. Which of the following phases of drug approval produces inconclusive therapeutic results?

    a. Clinical phase trials

    b. New drug application

    c. Preclinical investigation

    d. Postmarketing surveillance

22. In the drug approval process, what is the purpose of the postmarketing surveillance stage?

    a. Completion of laboratory tests on human cells

    b. Small clinical trials on volunteers

    c. Animal and human drug trials

    d. Survey for harmful effects in a large human population

23. What is the purpose of the Prescription Drug User Fee Act?

    a. To regulate use of dietary supplements

    b. To provide yearly user fees to the FDA

    c. To charge a lower fee to those who are chronically ill

    d. To allow elders to use drugs with greater freedom

24. Which of the following statements best describes an advantage of prescription drugs over OTC drugs?

    a. OTC drugs do not require a physician's order.

    b. Prescription drugs ensure that harmful reactions, ineffective treatment, or a progressive disease state will not occur.

    c. Only patients authorized to receive prescription drugs will take these medications.

    d. The nurse can maximize therapy by ordering the amount and frequency to be dispensed.

25. Determining the usefulness of plant extracts, herbs, vitamins, minerals and dietary supplements for use in the American public is the role of:

    a. Center for Drug Evaluation and Research (CDER)

    b. Center for Biologics Evaluation and Research (CBER)

    c. Center for Food Safety and Applied Nutrition (CFSAN)

    d. National Center for Complementary and Alternative Medicine (NCCAM)

26. Which act represents the FDA's effort to enhance the use of bioinformation for improvement of candidate medical products including the fields of genomics and proteonomics, imaging, and bioinformatics?

    a. Bioterrorism Act

    b. FDA Amendments Act

    c. FDA Food Safety Modernization Act

    d. FDA's Critical Path Initiative

27. The action established in 1997, by the FDA to monitor drugs with a potential for causing death or serious injury was:

    a. Black box warnings

    b. Postmarketing surveillance

    c. Health care reform

    d. FDA Drug Modernization Act

CASE STUDY APPLICATIONS

28. A male patient has a problem with mild constipation. This symptom has just occurred and does not seem to be related to a major illness. He has considered trying OTC drugs such as Ex-Lax or Metamucil. He is also considering some natural alternative therapies.

    a. Using knowledge of pharmacology, what teaching plan would the nurse implement for the patient?

    b. What nursing history is important when answering the patient's questions?

29. A female patient reports to the nurse that she is experiencing a drug reaction. She states that she may have taken a generic medication that does not meet the standard for all pharmaceutical products.

    a. What assessment data are essential in the initial phase of the nurse–patient relationship with the patient?

    b. What would the nurse teach the patient about drug regulations and standards?

CHAPTER 2

DRUG CLASSES AND SCHEDULES

FILL IN THE BLANK

From the textbook, find the correct word(s) to complete the statement(s).

1. With _____ classifications, drugs are organized on the basis of their usefulness in treating a particular disorder.

2. Drugs organized by _____ classifications are categorized based on how they produce their effects in the body.

3. A _____ drug is the original, well-understood drug model from which other drugs in a particular class have been developed.

4. The three types of drug names are _____, _____, and _____ names.

5. The description given to a drug by the International Union of Pure and Applied Chemistry (IUPAC) is its _____ name.

6. Drugs with more then one active ingredient are called _____.

7. One of the main arguments against substituting generic drugs for brand name drugs is differences in _____.

8. A subdiscipline that deals with decisions relative to proper drug choices is the field of _____.

Adams/Holland, *Student Workbook and Resource Guide for Pharmacology for Nurses* 4th Edition
© 2014 by Pearson Education, Inc.

MATCHING

For questions 9 through 12, match the concept in column I with the concept in column II.

Column I	Column II
9. _____ pharmacologic classification	a. antihypertensive
10. _____ therapeutic classification	b. calcium channel blocker
11. _____ generic name	c. brand name
12. _____ trade name	d. active ingredients

MULTIPLE CHOICE

13. What is the key to the therapeutic classification of a drug?

    a. Link the disorder to the drug's clinical usefulness

    b. Clearly state what a drug does chemically

    c. Evaluate the body system affected by the drug

    d. Identify tissue changes that result after the medication is absorbed

14. A drug's trade name is assigned by whom?

    a. FDA

    b. U.S. Adopted Name Council

    c. Developing pharmaceutical company

    d. International Union of Pure and Applied Chemistry

15. Which of the following statements best explains why a drug would be placed on the negative drug formulary list?

    a. Absorption of the drug affects drug action.

    b. Distribution of the drug to the target cells is prolonged.

    c. Bioavailability is different and affects drug uptake.

    d. Generic drug bioavailability is different from the brand name and affects patient outcomes.

16. Why is a drug classified as a scheduled drug?

    a. The drug can cause dependency.

    b. Alcohol is part of the drug composition.

    c. Generic and brand name drugs have different bioavailability.

    d. The generic drug company still has exclusive rights to production.

17. Which of the following substances requires classification as a scheduled drug?

    a. Vodka

    b. Morphine

    c. Benadryl

    d. Cigarettes

18. Which of the following schedule classifications has the highest potential for abuse?

    a. Schedule I

    b. Schedule II

    c. Schedule III

    d. Schedule IV

19. Which of the following schedule classifications has the sole purpose of use as a research agent?

    a. Schedule I

    b. Schedule II

    c. Schedule III

    d. Schedule IV

20. In the United States, what law or agency restricts the use of controlled substances?

    a. FDA

    b. U.S. Pharmacopeia

    c. U.S. Adopted Name Council

    d. Controlled Substances Act

21. If for a particular drug there are no controlled studies in women or if studies in women and animals are not available to establish risk in pregnancy, the FDA classification is:

    a. Category A

    b. Category B

    c. Category C

    d. Category D

CASE STUDY APPLICATION

22. The nurse is giving a hospitalized patient her morning medications. The patient asks the nurse why she is giving the generic form of acetaminophen instead of the trade product, Tylenol. The patient asks if there is a difference between trade and generic products.

    a. What is the nurse's best reply?

    b. The patient also asks if Tylenol is a controlled substance. What is the nurse's best reply?

CHAPTER 3

PRINCIPLES OF DRUG ADMINISTRATION

FILL IN THE BLANK

From the textbook, find the correct word(s) to complete the statement(s).

1. The _____ route means the nurse will administer the drug to the patient by mouth, under the tongue, or into the rectum.

2. When the nurse places a drug directly onto the skin or associated membranes, this is referred to as the _____ route.

3. The traditional _____ _____ of drug administration form the operational basis for the safe delivery of medications.

4. Drugs swallowed, chewed, or slowly dissolved in the mouth are referred to as _____ medications.

5. _____ administration involves placing drugs under the tongue.

6. _____ and _____ are examples of rectal administration methods.

7. The most common method of drug delivery is the _____ route.

8. Drugs are injected directly into the muscle in the _____ route.

9. One popular method for delivering drugs across the skin at a slow steady rate is the _____ patch.

10. _____, _____, and _____ type drug delivery methods are useful in treating respiratory and reproductive ailments.

Adams/Holland, *Student Workbook and Resource Guide for Pharmacology for Nurses* 4th Edition
© 2014 by Pearson Education, Inc.

MATCHING

For questions 11 through 19, match the specific drug delivery method in column I with its general route in column II.

Column I	Column II
11. _____ rectal	a. enteral
12. _____ intravenous (IV)	b. parenteral
13. _____ intramuscular (IM)	c. topical
14. _____ oral (PO)	
15. _____ transmucosal	
16. _____ subcutaneous (SC or SQ)	
17. _____ transdermal	
18. _____ sublingual	
19. _____ intradermal	

MULTIPLE CHOICE

20. Which of the following statements about dissolution should the nurse consider correct?

    a. The shorter the dissolution time, the more delayed is the onset of action.

    b. Water, taken in combination with solid drug formulations, is meant only to help dissolve the drugs.

    c. The process of dissolving solid drugs is dissolution.

    d. Dissolution time is only important for dissolving drugs prior to drug administration.

21. Which of the following is considered a standing order?

    a. STAT

    b. prn

    c. NOW

    d. ASAP

22. Of the following patients, which would be appropriate for rectal administration?

    a. Unconscious patient

    b. Patient experiencing nausea or vomiting

    c. Infant who cannot swallow pills

    d. All of the above

23. Which of the following methods is NOT a parenteral method of drug administration and avoids the first-pass effect in the liver?

    a. Oral

    b. Intravenous

    c. Intramuscular

    d. Sublingual

24. Which of the following is a major advantage of IV drug administration?

    a. The duration of drug action can be easily controlled.

    b. It is relatively free from the possibility of harmful effects.

    c. A precise concentration of drug can be administered into the bloodstream.

    d. The onset of drug action can be easily controlled.

25. What is a disadvantage of subcutaneous drug administration?

    a. The final drug concentration within the bloodstream is unpredictable.

    b. Drugs cannot be confined to a precise location.

    c. For safety reasons, patients must be conscious when they receive a subcutaneous injection.

    d. Pain, swelling, or infection may occur if proper precautions are not taken.

26. If rapid onset of action is critical, which of the following routes would the nurse choose?

    a. Intravenous

    b. Intramuscular

    c. Sublingual

    d. Rectal

27. Which of the following drug administration methods would the nurse use for the tuberculin test with purified protein derivative (PPD)?

    a. Topical

    b. Intradermal

    c. Subcutaneous

    d. Intramuscular

28. Implants are generally administered by which drug administration method?

    a. Intradermal

    b. Subcutaneous

    c. Intraperitoneal

    d. Intramuscular

29. Which of the following intravenous drug administration methods might be used to instill adjunct medications, such as antibiotics and analgesics, over a short time period?

    a. Intraperitoneal

    b. Intermittent infusion

    c. Large-volume infusion

    d. IV bolus administration

30. Which of the following is true about the physical properties of drugs?

    a. Substances that are able to dissolve in lipids (fats) are called hydrophilic.

    b. Hydrophobic drugs mix well in the bloodstream but move less efficiently across body membranes.

c. Drugs with lipid properties mix well with components of cellular membranes.

d. All of the above are correct.

31. Which of the following statements is true about IV infusions?

    a. Single drug doses are generally administered over a shorter period of time.

    b. A flow regulator is always used to regulate drug flow.

    c. Quick delivery of IV drugs is not possible with IV infusion.

    d. Drug doses are generally administered by way of a syringe and needle.

32. What is the deepest skin layer superficial to subcutaneous tissue?

    a. Epidermis

    b. Dermis

    c. Hypodermis

    d. Muscular layer

33. Which of the following statements is true regarding topical drug applications?

    a. For a local effect, it is necessary to keep drugs from penetrating the skin barrier.

    b. Liquids and liquid mixtures are the most effective physical compositions for topical drug therapy.

    c. In some cases, it is desirable for topical drugs to enter the systemic circulation.

    d. All of the above are correct.

34. What is the most common type of drug formulation for eye and ear medications?

    a. Salves

    b. Ointments

    c. Drops

    d. Sprays

CASE STUDY APPLICATIONS

35. In some cases, many different formulations are available, giving patients more than one option for drug therapy. Birth control is an example. Patients may take birth control pills, receive injections, or take medication via transdermal patches or vaginal inserts. Each method has advantages and disadvantages. Consider a situation in which the nurse's patient, a 34-year-old working mother, has an active lifestyle and needs a reliable and effective means of birth control.

    a. What assessment data should be gathered?

    b. Outline the patient teaching necessary to help this patient make the best choice.

36. An elderly man presents with a complaint of nausea and diarrhea. After a thorough assessment, the health care provider determines that medication might help relieve some of these symptoms and requests the nurse to administer the medication.

    a. In planning drug administration routes, what would the nurse recommend for this patient and why?

    b. How will the nurse evaluate effectiveness of this route of administration?

CHAPTER 4

PHARMACOKINETICS

FILL IN THE BLANK

From the textbook, find the correct word(s) to complete the statement(s).

1. The four main categories used to group processes relating to pharmacokinetics are _____, _____, _____, and _____.

2. The brain and placenta have barriers that prevent some medications from gaining access through normal circulation. These are the _____ and _____ barriers.

3. _____ is a process whereby most medications are deactivated when passing through the liver.

4. A mechanism called the _____ _____ decreases the activity of most medications traveling through the liver.

5. _____ is a process involving the movement of a substance from its site of administration across body membranes to circulating fluids.

6. The rate of _____ determines how quickly the drug disintegrates and disperses into simpler forms.

7. Medications are removed from the body by the process of _____.

8. _____ _____ is the plasma level of a medication that will result in serious adverse effects for the patient.

9. The plasma drug concentration between the minimum effective concentration and the toxic concentration is called the _____ _____ of the drug.

10. A _____ dose is a higher amount of drug given to "prime" the patient's bloodstream with a level of drug sufficient to quickly induce a therapeutic response.

Adams/Holland, *Student Workbook and Resource Guide for Pharmacology for Nurses* 4th Edition
© 2014 by Pearson Education, Inc.

MATCHING

For questions 11 through 14, match the factors affecting absorption in column I with the absorption/distribution rates shown in column II.

Column I	Column II
11. _____ absence of food in the digestive tract	a. faster absorption/distribution rate
12. _____ binding of a drug to plasma proteins	b. slower absorption/distribution rate
13. _____ ability to mix with lipids	
14. _____ larger drug particle	

MULTIPLE CHOICE

15. What is the process of moving a medication from its site of administration across one or more body membranes?

    a. Absorption

    b. Distribution

    c. Metabolism

    d. Excretion

16. What process describes how drugs are transported in the body?

    a. Absorption

    b. Distribution

    c. Metabolism

    d. Excretion

17. What term describes how much of a drug is available to produce a biologic response?

    a. Volume of distribution

    b. Rate of elimination

    c. Bioavailability

    d. Half-life ($t_{1/2}$)

18. The type of drug-drug interaction where there is a *potentiated* (more than total) effect is called:

    a. Addition

    b. Synergism

    c. Antagonism

    d. Displacement

19. Which of the following refers to the removal of larger drug metabolites from the bloodstream to the urine?

    a. Filtration

    b. Reabsorption

    c. Secretion

    d. Recirculation

20. Which of the following is a true statement regarding the half-life of a medication?

    a. The greater the half-life, the longer the drug takes to be excreted.

    b. The longer the half-life of a drug, the shorter is the duration of drug action.

    c. Half-life and therapeutic range are terms that may be used interchangeably.

    d. When one knows the onset of drug action, one knows the half-life of a drug.

21. When a drug is highly bound to protein complexes, what is the effect on the patient?

    a. Drugs bound to protein are not available for distribution to body tissues.

    b. Highly bound drugs reach their target cells very quickly.

    c. These drugs cross the blood–brain barrier in minutes.

    d. Protein binding makes the drug more water soluble.

22. Which of the following routes of medication delivery do NOT bypass the first-pass effect?

    a. Rectal

    b. Sublingual

    c. Oral

    d. Parenteral

23. Which of the following body systems, if altered, could dramatically affect pharmacokinetics?

    a. Integumentary

    b. Musculoskeletal

    c. Sensory

    d. Renal

24. After drug therapy has been discontinued, what processes in the body contribute to the drug's presence in the body for several more weeks?

    a. Enterohepatic recirculation

    b. Integumentary elimination

    c. Respiratory elimination

    d. Renal excretion

CASE STUDY APPLICATIONS

25. A male patient is anxious and has not been able to sleep well for several weeks. He is moderately obese and has a history of hypertension and diabetes. After examination, the health care provider agrees to provide this patient with a drug to treat anxiety.

   a. What assessment data support the fact that drug distribution could be a problem for this patient?

   b. How will the nurse evaluate the effectiveness of the drugs used to treat anxiety?

   c. What is the primary site for excretion of this patient's medications and, therefore, the system that must be consistently evaluated by the nurse?

26. A 60-year-old man has been abusing alcohol for years. He appears to have no major medical problems. He has been admitted to an outpatient setting for a diagnostic evaluation of his bowel by colonoscopy.

   a. What elements of his history would alert the nurse to possible problems with pharmacokinetics?

   b. What interventions might the nurse expect during the medication phase of this procedure?

   c. What system(s) should the nurse assess following the delivery of any medications for this patient?

CHAPTER 5

PHARMACODYNAMICS

FILL IN THE BLANK

From the textbook, find the correct word(s) to complete the statement(s).

1. _____ deals with how medications affect body responses.

2. The classic theory about the cellular mechanism by which most medications produce a response is called the _____ theory.

3. _____ refers to a drug's strength at a particular concentration or dose, whereas _____ refers to the effectiveness of a drug in producing a more intense response as the concentration is increased.

4. A _____ _____ curve is a graphical representation of the actual number of patients responding to a drug action at different doses.

5. The median effective dose (ED_{50}) is the dose required to produce a specific therapeutic response in _____% of a group of patients.

6. The median lethal dose (LD_{50}) is the dose of drug that will be _____ in 50% of a group of animals.

7. A drug's _____ _____ offers the nurse practical information on the safety of a drug.

8. A drug that is more potent will produce a therapeutic effect at a _____ dose, compared to another drug in the same class.

9. By observing and measuring the _____ _____ _____ or the patient's response obtained at different doses of the drug, one can see the different phases of drug relief.

10. _____ often compete with agonists for the receptor binding sites.

Adams/Holland, *Student Workbook and Resource Guide for Pharmacology for Nurses* 4th Edition
© 2014 by Pearson Education, Inc.

MATCHING

For questions 11 through 15, match the factors influencing drug effectiveness in column I with the area of pharmacokinetics or pharmacodynamics in column II.

Column I

11. _____ concentration (dose) of an administered drug

12. _____ presence of food in the digestive tract

13. _____ frequency of drug dosing

14. _____ age of the patient

15. _____ kidney disease

Column II

a. pharmacokinetics

b. pharmacodynamics

MULTIPLE CHOICE

16. Which of the following best explains the pharmacodynamic phase of drug administration?

    a. The way the drug is absorbed, distributed, and eliminated from the body

    b. Drug action and the relationship between drug concentration and body responses

    c. Movement of substances from the site of administration across body membranes

    d. First-pass effect, which determines the frequency of dosing

17. The nurse is giving a drug with which she is unfamiliar. The nurse checks the drug guide and determines that the average dose for the drug is 100 mg/day. Which of the following statements best explains what that means to the nurse?

    a. The amount (100 mg) will be the effective dosing for about 50% of the population.

    b. The amount (100 mg) is the normal dose and it should be given twice per day.

    c. Few patients will respond to the 100-mg dose without side effects.

    d. Most patients will have a reaction if given more than 100 mg/day.

18. The nurse is explaining to a patient the concept of drug potency. Which of the following statements best explains the concept?

    a. "If you are told to consider equivalent drugs to control thyroid problems, the drug with the lowest milligram weight is the most potent."

    b. "A 100-mg dose is a more potent drug dosing than a 50-mg dose."

    c. "Dosing has nothing to do with potency. The site of injection is the most important part of dosing theory."

    d. "Your size and weight determine drug potency."

19. When drug molecules bind with cell receptors, what occurs?

    a. Pharmacologic effects of agonism or antagonism occur.

    b. Pharmacogenetics occurs quickly.

    c. The therapeutic index is increased.

    d. Potency of the drug is altered.

20. The pharmacist tells the nurse that a drug has a high therapeutic index. Which of the following statements best reflects the nurse's understanding of that statement?

    a. Phase I of the dose–response curve would be low.

    b. It is therapeutic to give this drug once per day.

    c. It would take a big error in dosing to create a lethal dose for this patient.

    d. The nurse should be very careful—there are a lot of receptors that are sensitive to this drug.

21. Which pharmacologic principles will guide the nurse's practice?

    a. Future medications may be customized to match the patient's genetic makeup.

    b. If the nurse understands potency and efficacy, the nurse can compare medications.

    c. As the therapeutic index increases, the safety of the drug increases.

    d. All of the above are correct.

22. The nurse is reviewing the terms *efficacy* and *potency* with a patient who is receiving medications for cancer. What statement is most correct?

    a. "You need to be most interested in the number of milligrams the medication is going to provide. This is called potency."

    b. "The number of cancer cells killed is called efficacy. You are most interested in efficacy in the treatment of your disease."

    c. "Your cancer is going to require that the fewest numbers of receptors be affected. So, concentrate on potency."

    d. "Cancer is so affected by genetics. It is best to ask questions about dose and drug reactions, not efficacy."

23. The nurse hears in a report that a patient had an idiosyncratic reaction to a medication. Which of the following statements best explains what happened to the patient?

    a. No response, good or bad, was seen 24 hours after delivery of the medication.

    b. Drug-to-drug interaction occurred and less medication was needed.

    c. An unpredictable and unexplained drug reaction occurred.

    d. An antagonist reaction occurred at the receptor level.

24. Which statement best describes antagonists?

    a. They are sometimes referred to as facilitators of drug action.

    b. They can only produce an effect by interacting with receptors.

    c. They inhibit or block the action of agonist drugs.

    d. All of the above are correct.

25. The nurse is giving two drugs to a patient with a heart problem. One drug works at the $beta_1$-adrenergic receptor and the other works at the $beta_2$ receptor. Which of the following statements bests explains how that can be possible?

    a. This is an example of potency and must be questioned.

    b. The graded dose response is the best explanation for this order.

    c. Lethal dose is determined on preclinical trials of beta-receptor drugs.

    d. The drugs are fine-tuned and can affect the different beta-receptor types in specific ways.

CHAPTER 5 / Pharmacodynamics   **19**

CASE STUDY APPLICATIONS

26. A patient with a history of severe migraines is taking an analgesic that is classified as an agonist/antagonist. The patient has not asked for the analgesic for 3 hours.

    a. What nursing assessment would the nurse perform before giving this analgesic?

    b. What nursing diagnosis would the nurse consider before giving this analgesic?

    c. What questions would the nurse ask if the migraine headaches are not relieved within 15 minutes?

27. The nurse is a nurse working with patients in an infectious disease clinic. Several of the patients are complaining that their wound infections are not healing quickly enough. The nurse reviews their medical records.

    a. What information is the nurse looking for related to pharmacotherapy?

    b. What outcomes would the nurse expect to measure for the patient in a wound management clinic?

    c. What evaluation would support the nurse's recommendation for a medication change?

Adams/Holland, *Student Workbook and Resource Guide for Pharmacology for Nurses* 4th Edition
© 2014 by Pearson Education, Inc.

CHAPTER 6

THE NURSING PROCESS IN PHARMACOLOGY

FILL IN THE BLANK

From the textbook, find the correct word(s) to complete the statement(s).

1. _____ are clinical judgments of a patient's actual or potential health problem that is within the nurse's scope of practice to address.

2. The _____ phase of the nursing process is used to determine whether or not the therapeutic effects of the drug were achieved.

3. Nurses use their skills in _____ during the interview to collect data that are denied or downplayed.

4. The _____ _____ is a systematic method of problem solving that forms the foundation for nursing practice.

Adams/Holland, *Student Workbook and Resource Guide for Pharmacology for Nurses* 4th Edition
© 2014 by Pearson Education, Inc.

MATCHING

For questions 5 through 11, match the description in column I with the nursing process step in column II.

Column I

5. _____ first step in the nursing process

6. _____ data that include what the patient says

7. _____ data gathered through diagnostic sources

8. _____ provide the basis for planning patient care

9. _____ objective measures of goals

10. _____ links interventions to established outcomes

11. _____ assessment of goals and outcomes

Column II

a. evaluation

b. intervention

c. nursing diagnoses

d. objective data

e. subjective data

f. assessment

g. outcomes

h. planning

MULTIPLE CHOICE

12. A male patient has just returned from surgery. The nurse is taking the patient's vital signs, checking his incision site, and determining if he is in pain. What step of the nursing process is the nurse using?

    a. Evaluation

    b. Planning

    c. Assessment

    d. Intervention

13. A male patient has begun to complain of pain in his incision site. The nurse is administering morphine sulfate 2 mg IV. What step of the nursing process is the nurse using?

    a. Evaluation

    b. Planning

    c. Assessment

    d. Intervention

14. A male patient has inquired about the physical therapy he will be receiving to regain his mobility after his knee replacement surgery. The nurse will interact with physical therapy to coordinate his plan of care. What step of the nursing process is the nurse using?

    a. Evaluation

    b. Planning

    c. Assessment

    d. Intervention

15. A male patient received physical therapy and has regained his mobility after his knee replacement surgery. The nurse interacts with physical therapy to determine if the patient is ready to be discharged from the skilled unit. What step of the nursing process is the nurse using?

    a. Evaluation

    b. Planning

    c. Assessment

    d. Intervention

16. A female patient is complaining of pain in her right hip. The nurse records in the medical record that the patient reported pain on walking and that it was worse at night. What type of information has the nurse gathered?

    a. Objective data

    b. Subjective data

    c. Outcomes

    d. Goals

17. A female patient is complaining of pain in her right hip. The nurse has assessed the area and has found swelling, redness, and open areas, and there is a history of trauma to the hip. What type of information has the nurse gathered?

    a. Objective data

    b. Subjective data

    c. Outcomes

    d. Goals

18. A female patient is complaining of pain in her right hip. The nurse has assessed the area and has found swelling, redness, and open areas, and there is a history of trauma to the hip. This information will be used to compare with assessment information gathered following surgery. What type of information has the nurse gathered?

    a. Objective data

    b. Subjective data

    c. Outcomes

    d. Baseline data

19. A female patient is recovering from a fracture of the right hip. The interdisciplinary team has established a schedule of physical therapy for her. She will ambulate using a walker with the assist of one member of the team for 50 ft three times a day for 1 week, to be increased to 100 ft three times a day for 2 weeks, then to be changed to a quad cane and stand by assistance for 2 weeks and then discharged to home. What type of information has been presented?

    a. Evaluation

    b. Goals

    c. Baseline data

    d. Objective data

20. A female patient is recovering from a fracture of the right hip. The interdisciplinary team has established a schedule of physical therapy for her. She is ambulating using a quad cane without assistance. It has been established she is ready to be discharged to her home. What type of information has been presented?

    a. Outcomes

    b. Planning

    c. Baseline data

    d. Subjective data

21. Using the information in question 20, select the priority nursing diagnosis for the patient.

    a. *Pain* related to hip fracture, as evidenced by complaints of pain with ambulation

    b. *Immobility* related to hip fracture, as evidenced by inability to stand or ambulate without assistance

    c. Readiness for enhanced self health management related to impending discharge to home

    d. *Risk for Impaired Skin Integrity* related to immobility from hip fracture

22. What is the priority factor in establishing a plan of care for a patient who will be on a routine antihypertensive medication at home?

    a. Patient education on adverse effects of the medication

    b. Risk for noncompliance

    c. Arranging for the drug to be delivered

    d. Teaching the patient to take own blood pressure to ensure therapeutic effects

23. What factor established from the patient's health history would suggest the greatest potential for noncompliance with the medication regimen?

    a. Male

    b. Female

    c. Elderly

    d. Live in an urban area

24. The nurse is developing goals and outcomes for a female patient who is being discharged today following recent abdominal surgery. One key element regarding these goals is that they:

    a. should be patient oriented.

    b. should be nurse oriented.

    c. should include at least three outcomes.

    d. should not be seen by the patient prior to discharge.

MAKING CONNECTIONS

25. All drugs have more than one:

    a. name.

    b. active ingredient.

    c. generic name.

    d. indication.

26. How do therapeutic drugs differ from foods, household products, and cosmetics?

    a. Only therapeutic drugs can induce a biologic response.

    b. Food, household products, and cosmetics are not designed for the treatment of disease and suffering.

c. Drugs may not be considered as substances that contribute to the body's normal activities.

d. Drugs are narrowly defined.

27. Which method is used for fast delivery of a drug to the cerebrospinal fluid?

a. Intraperitoneal

b. Intrathecal

c. Epidural

d. Transmucosal

28. Which term describes how much of a drug is available to produce a response?

a. Volume of distribution

b. Rate of elimination

c. Bioavailability

d. Half-life

29. What is the process of moving a drug from its site of administration across one or more body membranes to circulating fluids?

a. Absorption

b. Metabolism

c. Distribution

d. Excretion

CASE STUDY APPLICATIONS

30. A 15-year-old girl has just been diagnosed with type 1 diabetes mellitus. She has presented to the emergency department on three occasions with blood glucose of over 400. She refuses to follow her prescribed diet and insulin regimen. She states, "My friends and classmates think that I am weird when I don't eat what they do and when I have to give myself a shot." The nurse must remember certain factors related to this age group when establishing the plan of care.

a. What special consideration should the nurse give to this patient in regard to patient teaching?

b. What would be the nurse's priority nursing diagnosis?

31. A 35-year-old female Hispanic migrant worker who does not speak or understand English presents to the emergency department with severe abdominal pain and rigidity in the right lower quadrant. The nurse is to take the health history and establish a plan of care.

a. What would be the nurse's priority intervention in this patient's plan of care?

b. What barriers would the nurse expect to encounter when establishing her plan of care?

32. A 25-year-old male patient with a history of substance abuse has been admitted to the nurse's area after receiving critical injuries in a car wreck. He is now recovering and has moved to the acute ward from ICU. The nurse establishing his plan of care may encounter barriers in regard to his recovery.

a. What effects could his substance abuse have on his recovery?

b. What goals and outcomes will the nurse establish for this patient?

CHAPTER 7

MEDICATION ERRORS
AND RISK REDUCTION

FILL IN THE BLANK

From the textbook, find the correct word(s) to complete the statement(s).

1. A medication error is any _____ event that may cause or lead to inappropriate medication use or cause _____ _____ while the medication is in the control of the health care professional, patient, or consumer.

2. Unexpected occurrences involving death or serious physical or psychological injury are called _____.

3. The process of "keeping track" of patient's medications as they transfer from one health care provider to another is called _____ _____.

4. Incomplete orders should be _____ with the prescriber before the drug is _____.

5. In the home setting, the drug most frequently associated with medication errors is _____.

Adams/Holland, *Student Workbook and Resource Guide for Pharmacology for Nurses* 4th Edition
© 2014 by Pearson Education, Inc.

MATCHING

For questions 6 through 9, match the definition in column I with its key term in column II.

Column I

6. _____ To observe or record relevant physiological or psychological signs

7. _____ Includes cardiovascular and respiratory support (e.g., CPR, defibrillation, intubation)

8. _____ Impairment of the physical, emotional, or psychological function or structure of the body and/or pain resulting therefrom

9. _____ May include change in therapy or active medical/surgical treatment

Column II

a. Harm

b. Monitoring

c. Intervention

d. Intervention Necessary to Sustain Life

MULTIPLE CHOICE

10. Assessment is the most important step of the nursing process in preventing medication errors by which of the following?

    a. Having the patient state the outcome of the medication

    b. Obtaining allergy and medication history information

    c. Advising the patient to question the nurse about medications

    d. Planning the correct times for the patient to take medications

11. Which best describes the reporting of medication errors?

    a. Is voluntary in ethical nursing practice

    b. Must be kept confidential in nursing practice

    c. Is an optional act on the part of the nurse

    d. Is responsible and accountable by the nurse

12. Nurses should know that a common type of medication error is which of the following?

    a. Giving the wrong drug

    b. Giving the wrong dose

    c. Giving a drug by the wrong route of administration

    d. All of the above

13. The nurse should NOT use which of the following abbreviations because it has been found to result in medication errors?

    a. tid

    b. bid

    c. qd

    d. prn

14. All of the following are true regarding medication errors EXCEPT:

    a. they are only documented if they cause harm, or potential harm, to the patient.

    b. they can be reduced by having the patient fill all prescriptions at one pharmacy.

    c. they may be reported anonymously to the FDA.

    d. they can be reduced by using medication reconciliation.

15. A nurse has given an incorrect dose of a medication. She follows the agency protocol by completing an incident report and discussing the incident with the risk manager. The primary purpose of following this procedure for reporting errors is to:

    a. determine the competence of the nurse.

    b. prevent future medication errors.

    c. determine who is to blame.

    d. gather information for risk management procedures.

16. Morphine every 4 hours is ordered for a patient with terminal cancer who is experiencing severe pain. The nurse records that the patient's respirations are 12 per minute and administers the medication as ordered. Twenty minutes later, the patient develops respiratory arrest and dies. Which of the following statements provides the most accurate description of the nurse's dilemma?

    a. The nurse should have notified the health care provider for a clarification of the order.

    b. The nurse should have reassessed the patient in 30 minutes to determine further nursing action.

    c. The nurse should have withheld a dose of the medication because the patient's respirations were too slow.

    d. The nurse's intention was to alleviate pain, using a reasonable and prudent manner.

17. What should a nurse document, if a medication error occurs?

    a. Document routine assessments and observations in the patient's chart.

    b. Complete an incident report and place a copy in the patient's chart.

    c. Document who was to blame for the medication error.

    d. Document all nursing interventions taken to protect patient safety on the patient's chart.

18. As the nurses hands the medication cimetidine (Tagamet) to the patient, the patient states, "Thank you. This is the pill that neutralizes the acid in my stomach, so that I don't get heartburn." The nurse will take which step in the nursing process?

    a. Assessment

    b. Planning

    c. Intervention

    d. Evaluation

19. While administering the 10 a.m. medications, the nurse discovers that the 6 a.m. intravenous dose was still hanging and never infused. What should be the nurse's first action?

    a. Document these findings on the patient's chart.

    b. Notify the primary health care provider.

    c. Complete an incident report.

    d. Begin the first infusion.

Adams/Holland, *Student Workbook and Resource Guide for Pharmacology for Nurses* 4th Edition
© 2014 by Pearson Education, Inc.

20. The physician approaches the nurse while she is preparing a medication. The nurse asks the physician to come back in 10 minutes. This is an example of which step in the nursing process?

    a. Assessment

    b. Planning

    c. Intervention

    d. Evaluation

21. When the nurse hands the patient his morning medications, the patient says, "There's a yellow tablet in the cup. The doctor must have ordered a new pill." Which of the following responses is the best reply?

    a. "Let me check with the pharmacist to see if that pill is appropriate for you."

    b. "Yes. It is the right medication. Would you like some water to take with your pills?"

    c. "Let me check the doctor's orders and the medication administration record."

    d. "Would you like me to check the doctor's orders?"

22. A nurse, who is doing telephone triage for an outpatient clinic, receives a call from a 76-year-old woman who is concerned because she has not had a bowel movement in 3 days and reports that "her stomach really hurts." Which of the following responses is correct?

    a. The nurse suggests that she eat foods high in fiber and drink some prune juice.

    b. The nurse suggests that she take a gentle laxative and drink more fluids.

    c. The nurse suggests that she call her primary care provider and have a more complete assessment.

    d. The nurse suggests that she use a glycerin suppository.

23. A nurse administers a health care provider's order for 150 mg of medication, when the usual dosage is 75 mg. When the nurse manager discusses the incident with the nurse, the nurse states that the dosage administered is what the health care provider ordered. What should the nurse manager tell the nurse?

    a. "It is not your fault. The provider ordered the wrong dosage."

    b. "This was a serious error. You must have misread the order."

    c. "It is your responsibility to know the correct dosage. If the dosage seemed incorrect, it was your responsibility to call the health care provider."

    d. "Did you ask the health care provider why the dosage was higher than usual?"

24. The nurse is preparing to administer a dose of an enteric-coated tablet to a patient. The patient states that he is unable to swallow a pill. What is the correct action by the nurse?

    a. Instruct the patient to place the tablet on the back of his tongue and give him large amounts of water immediately.

    b. Leave the tablet at the bedside and instruct the patient to take it later.

    c. Crush the tablet and mix it in applesauce. Then, administer the tablet in applesauce to the patient.

    d. Return to the medication room with the medication and notify the health care provider.

25. Tetracycline 500 mg bid by mouth has been ordered for a 36-year-old forest ranger who has been diagnosed with Lyme disease. He tells the nurse that antibiotics often give him indigestion, so the nurse gives him a glass of milk to take with his medication. How could this medication error be avoided?

   a. He should be receiving 500 mg four times a day.

   b. This medication should be given intravenously to be effective.

   c. Sulfa drugs are more effective in the initial treatment of Lyme disease.

   d. Do not give drug with milk products because these inhibit absorption.

MAKING CONNECTIONS

26. Which federal agency is responsible for determining the effectiveness of all new drugs proposed each year?

   a. Food and Drug Administration (FDA)

   b. Drug Enforcement Agency (DEA)

   c. National Institutes of Health (NIH)

   d. United States Public Health Service (USPHS)

27. All opioids are assigned a schedule or classification by law. In which schedule will the nurse find morphine sulfate?

   a. Schedule I

   b. Schedule II

   c. Schedule III

   d. Schedule IV

28. What does it mean when a drug is classified as being teratogenic?

   a. It is safe for the mother in the first trimester of pregnancy.

   b. It is safe for the mother in the last trimester of pregnancy.

   c. Harmful effects on the fetus may occur at high doses.

   d. It is not safe for the fetus and may cause birth defects.

29. Which of the following is a normal change in physiology that occurs with aging?

   a. Absorption of drugs is more rapid.

   b. Cardiac output is higher, distributing drugs more rapidly.

   c. Hepatic function decreases, slowing drug metabolism.

   d. Immune function increases, reducing the need for prophylactic antibiotics.

30. Which legal agency deals with the enforcement of substance abuse laws?

   a. Food and Drug Administration (FDA)

   b. Drug Enforcement Agency (DEA)

   c. National Institutes of Health (NIH)

   d. None of the above

CASE STUDY APPLICATIONS

31. An older adult refuses an antihypertensive drug after breakfast. The nurse notes that this has happened 3 days in a row. The patient's blood pressure has risen 40 mmHg and the patient complains of an occipital headache.

    a. What step of the nursing process is utilized in this scenario? What type of data are described in this process?

    b. What steps could the nurse have taken to prevent this noncompliance with the drug regimen?

32. While preparing medications, the nurse notes that the patient has been receiving an anticoagulant daily but the order reads that it should be given every other day.

    a. What would be an appropriate nursing diagnosis for this patient?

    b. What nursing interventions would be included in the plan of care?

33. A 34-year-old woman, with a diagnosis of bipolar disorder, is admitted to the behavioral health unit and is reporting fine hand tremors, nausea, slurred speech, and dizziness. The medication that she has been taking is lithium carbonate (Eskalith) 300 mg bid and risperidone (Risperdal) 0.5 mg at 10 a.m. and at bedtime. Because it is time for the patient's next dose of lithium, the nurse administers the medication before proceeding with the nursing assessment. While gathering information for the assessment, the patient tells the nurse that she has recently been taking a diuretic because of fluid retention before her menstrual period.

    a. What further information and assessments are indicated at this time?

    b. Should the nurse have delayed the next dose and contacted the health care provider? Why?

    c. The health care provider orders an increase of lithium to 300 mg tid. What should the nurse do?

34. Ferrous sulfate is ordered at 10 a.m., 2 p.m., and 6 p.m. However, the patient is scheduled for physical therapy at 9 a.m. The nurse decides to give the medication at 8 a.m. with breakfast, since the nurse knows that administering iron supplements with food reduces gastric irritation. However, the medication is charted as if it were given at 10 a.m.

    a. Is this considered a medication error?

    b. What is the best way for the nurse to handle this situation?

CHAPTER 8

DRUG ADMINISTRATION THROUGHOUT THE LIFE SPAN

FILL IN THE BLANK

From the textbook, find the correct word(s) to complete the statement(s).

1. A term that characterizes the progressive increase in physical size is _____.

2. The functional changes in the physical, psychomotor, and cognitive capabilities of a person are called _____.

3. Considering the individual needs of the patient and caring for the whole person are called _____ care.

4. During pregnancy, weeks 1–2 are the _____ period, weeks 3–8 are the _____ period and weeks 9–40 are the _____ period.

5. By the third trimester of pregnancy, blood flow through the _____ is reduced by 40% to 50%, which may affect drug _____.

6. In older adults hepatic metabolism _____, which may require _____ drug dosages for this age group.

7. A substance that may produce permanent changes to an embryo or fetus is called a/an _____.

8. The taking of multiple drugs, or _____, in older adults increases the risk for drug interactions and adverse effects.

Adams/Holland, *Student Workbook and Resource Guide for Pharmacology for Nurses* 4th Edition
© 2014 by Pearson Education, Inc.

MATCHING

For questions 9 through 13, match the pregnancy categories in column I with their descriptions in column II.

Column I

9. _____ Category A

10. _____ Category B

11. _____ Category C

12. _____ Category D

13. _____ Category X

Column II

a. Studies in pregnant women have *not* shown an increased risk to the fetus during any trimester of pregnancy.

b. Animal studies *have* shown risks to the fetus and there are no well-controlled studies in pregnant women.

c. Studies in pregnant women have shown an increased risk to the fetus but the benefits of the drug may outweigh the potential risk.

d. Studies in animals or pregnant women *have* shown a significant risk to the fetus.

e. Animal studies have *not* shown a risk to the fetus; however, there are no well-controlled studies in pregnant women.

MULTIPLE CHOICE

14. During the first trimester of pregnancy, what is (are) the primary consideration(s) from a medical, nursing, and pharmacologic viewpoint?

   a. Assessing and evaluating each patient on an individual basis, so that mistaken beliefs can be clarified

   b. Safety of the patient and delivery of a healthy baby

   c. Evaluating the knowledge base of the mother in regard to growth and development

   d. A focus on reducing the physical discomforts of the mother

15. The nurse determines that the fetus is at the greatest risk for developmental and structural anomalies during which period?

   a. Preimplantation

   b. Embryonic

   c. Fetal

   d. Post-natal

16. During which period is there the greatest risk of a drug causing death of the growing embryo or fetus?

   a. Preimplantation

   b. Embryonic

   c. Fetal

   d. Post-natal

17. During a routine prenatal visit in her third trimester, a patient informs the nurse that she is smoking again because of a stressful situation at her job. The nurse counsels the patient on the increased risks to the fetus. Why are risks increased at this time?

   a. Blood flow to the placenta increases and placental vascular membranes become thinner.

   b. Drugs reaching the fetus have a reduced duration of action.

c. The fetus receives reduced amounts of substances from the maternal bloodstream.

d. Blood flow to the placenta decreases and placental vascular membranes become thicker.

18. The nurse correctly provides the following education to a breast-feeding patient:

    a. over-the-counter drugs may be safely taken.

    b. dietary supplements and herbal products may be safely taken.

    c. no dietary supplement, herb, or drug should be taken without approval of the health care provider.

    d. no prescription drugs should be taken.

19. What is the preferred site for administering an IM injection to an infant?

    a. Deltoid

    b. Dorsogluteal

    c. Gluteus maximus

    d. Vastus lateralis

20. When determining the correct method for calculating drug amount for infants, what must the nurse consider?

    a. Development of the immune system

    b. Development of the nervous system

    c. Age and size of the infant

    d. Infant's ability to swallow medications

21. When assessing risk factors, which age group must the nurse evaluate for a high risk for accidental poisoning from household products or drugs?

    a. School age

    b. Toddler

    c. Infant

    d. Preschool age

22. Before administering a drug to an older adult, the nurse should understand that the "average" dose may be affected by which of the following normal consequences of aging?

    a. Older adults have increased hepatic metabolism.

    b. Older adults have more rapid gastric motility.

    c. Older adults have reduced kidney function.

    d. Older adults have increased capacity for plasma protein binding.

23. During adolescence, the nurse assumes a key role in the patient's education in relationship to which of the following?

    a. Use of vitamins

    b. Use of herbal remedies

    c. Use of prescription medications

    d. Use of tobacco and illicit drugs

24. During which period of adulthood would the nurse expect to offer counseling regarding substance abuse and sexually transmitted diseases?

    a. Middle adulthood

    b. Young adulthood

    c. Older adulthood

    d. None of the above

25. During which period of adulthood would the nurse expect to offer counseling regarding positive lifestyle modifications?

    a. Middle adulthood

    b. Young adulthood

    c. Older adulthood

    d. None of the above

26. During which period of adulthood would the nurse expect to offer counseling regarding increased potential for adverse reactions to medications related to impaired physiologic and biochemical processes?

    a. Middle adulthood

    b. Young adulthood

    c. Older adulthood

    d. None of the above

27. The nurse knows that all of the following contribute to increased serum drug levels in the older adult EXCEPT:

    a. reduced total body water.

    b. decreased amounts of plasma proteins.

    c. increased hepatic metabolism.

    d. reduced renal excretion.

MAKING CONNECTIONS

28. Which branch of medicine deals with the general treatment of suffering and disease?

    a. Pharmacotherapeutics

    b. Pathophysiology

    c. Therapeutics

    d. Physiology

29. What does the prototype approach to drug therapy consider?

    a. Most popular drug for a particular disorder

    b. Most commonly used drug in a particular class

    c. Representative drug for how other drugs in a particular class work

    d. Drug of choice for a particular disorder

30. What is the most common type of drug formulation for eye and ear medications?

   a. Salves

   b. Ointments

   c. Drops

   d. Sprays

31. The nurse places a drug tablet between the patient's cheek and gum. What delivery route is being used for this patient?

   a. Buccal

   b. Sublingual

   c. Otic

   d. Subcutaneous

32. The nurse is administering Tylenol to reduce the fever of a child. What phase of the nursing process is the nurse using?

   a. Intervention

   b. Planning

   c. Outcome

   d. Assessment

CASE STUDY APPLICATIONS

33. A 19-year-old woman presents to the nurse's clinic 20 weeks pregnant. She has received no prenatal care, has a history of substance abuse, and admits to using tobacco, alcohol, and cocaine during her pregnancy. The nurse assesses for the potential of developmental anomalies for the fetus. The nurse also evaluates the potential for future complications if the substance abuse continues throughout the pregnancy.

   a. What are the potential anomalies in the fetus at the time of the visit?

   b. What are the potential complications to the pregnancy?

   c. State the rationale for the potential anomalies and complications.

34. A 52-year-old mother with two grown children, six grandchildren, and aging parents with various health problems presents to the nurse's clinic. The patient is married and her husband is disabled. She also has a full-time job and two part-time jobs. She is 50 pounds overweight and displays signs and symptoms of excessive stress. Evaluate the potential complications from this situation and emphasize changes in the nurse's patient education.

   a. What are middle-aged adults sometimes called?

   b. What options do these adults have to control their lifestyles?

   c. What health factors are often in place at this time in the life cycle?

35. A 72-year-old man presents with a variety of health problems. He is presently taking 14 different medications prescribed by four different health care providers. The nurse providing the patient education assesses the situation and determines the lifestyle changes that are necessary to ensure optimal health for this patient.

   a. Taking multiple drugs concurrently is known by what term?

   b. How does this action affect drug interactions and potential for adverse reactions?

   c. What areas should the nurse assess carefully in this patient's health history?

CHAPTER 9

PSYCHOSOCIAL, GENDER, AND CULTURAL INFLUENCES ON PHARMACOTHERAPY

FILL IN THE BLANK

From the textbook, find the correct word(s) to complete the statement(s).

1. The recipient of care must be regarded in a _____ context for health to be affected in a positive manner.

2. Strong spiritual or religious beliefs may greatly influence a person's _____ of their illness and their _____ _____ of treatment.

3. The ability of health care providers to provide effective care to people with diverse values, beliefs, and behaviors is called _____ _____.

4. The most obvious community-related negative influence on pharmacotherapy is _____ to health care.

5. The study of genetic variations that give rise to differences in the way patients handle medications is called _____.

Adams/Holland, *Student Workbook and Resource Guide for Pharmacology for Nurses* 4th Edition
© 2014 by Pearson Education, Inc.

MATCHING

For questions 6 through 10, match the definition in column I with its key term in column II.

Column I

6. _____ change in enzyme structure and function due to mutation in DNA

7. _____ study of human behavior within the context of groups and societies

8. _____ incorporates the capacity to love, to convey compassion, to enjoy life, and to find peace of mind and fulfillment

9. _____ community of people having a common history and similar genetic heritage

10. _____ beliefs, values, customs, and religious rituals shared by a group of people

Column II

a. culture

b. ethnic group

c. genetic polymorphism

d. psychology

e. sociology

f. spirituality

MULTIPLE CHOICE

11. Determining the patient's psychosocial history is essential in the initial assessment. It includes all of the following EXCEPT:

   a. religious beliefs.

   b. sexual practices.

   c. previous illnesses.

   d. use of alcohol, tobacco, or illegal drugs.

12. Which of the following patients is least likely to properly adhere to a medication regimen?

   a. The patient who trusts the nurse

   b. The patient who is aware of possible severe adverse effects associated with medications

   c. The patient who has high expectations regarding the results of taking medications

   d. The patient who has received limited information about medications

13. All of the following are true regarding genetic polymorphisms EXCEPT:

   a. they are often associated with specific ethnic groups.

   b. they are rare in the overall population.

   c. they can greatly impact the handling of medications by the body.

   d. they are more frequently seen in males.

14. Community-related variables that influence pharmacotherapy include all of the following EXCEPT:

   a. access to health care.

   b. alternative therapies.

   c. literacy.

   d. spiritual beliefs.

15. Which of the following statements by the nurse will help to ensure that the patient understands the instructions given?

    a. "Do you understand how to take your medications?"

    b. "You should take this drug at 8 a.m. and 8 p.m. Call the doctor if you have any problems."

    c. "Could you explain to me how you will take your medication at home?"

    d. "Here are some printed instructions on how to use your prescription medications."

16. What is the study of variations in drug response caused by mutations in DNA?

    a. Pharmacogenetics

    b. Eugenics

    c. Polymorphisms

    d. Acetylation

17. Which of the following drugs would have the least effect on a person of African American descent because of enzyme polymorphisms?

    a. Isoniazid

    b. Propranolol

    c. Codeine

    d. Warfarin

18. Which of the following statements regarding women's health is false?

    a. Women seek health care earlier than men.

    b. Women have a higher incidence of Alzheimer's disease than men.

    c. Women do not seek medical attention for potential cardiac problems as readily as men.

    d. Women do not like to use antihypertensive medications because of side effects.

19. Variables to consider when treating patients in different ethnic groups include all of the following EXCEPT:

    a. diet.

    b. alternative therapies.

    c. genetic differences.

    d. literacy.

20. Which of the following is the least useful method for supplying information regarding medication use at home to a patient who is functionally illiterate?

    a. Provide the patient with written information regarding the drug and its side effects.

    b. Provide the patient with diagrams and pictures showing how to use the inhaler.

    c. Instruct the patient's family about the inhaler at the same time the patient is receiving the information.

    d. Show the patient the inhaler each time it is administered and explain its use and side effects.

MAKING CONNECTIONS

21. Which of the following would the nurse find in a pharmacopoeia?

    a. Drugs of choice for specific disease

    b. Standards for assessing drug purity and strength

    c. Drug doses for pediatric and seriatric patients

    d. Results of clinical drug trials for newly approved medications

22. Which of the following drug schedules has the highest potential for abuse?

    a. Schedule I

    b. Schedule II

    c. Schedule III

    d. Schedule IV

23. Which phase of the nursing process includes the collection of information from the patient regarding prescription drugs currently being used, drug allergies, and the use of dietary supplements?

    a. Assessment

    b. Planning

    c. Intervention

    d. Evaluation

24. A female patient is in her first trimester of pregnancy. She has been told not to use a drug the physician called "teratogenic." She asks the nurse what this term means. The nurse tells her it is a substance:

    a. that could produce dependency.

    b. that could harm her developing fetus.

    c. used to induce labor.

    d. that cannot be obtained over the counter.

25. Which of the following drug delivery methods is an enteral method of drug delivery that avoids the first-pass effect in the liver?

    a. Oral

    b. Intrathecal

    c. Intramuscular

    d. Sublingual

CASE STUDY APPLICATIONS

26. A woman has come in for her monthly prenatal checkup. During the nurse's assessment she confides that her husband is an alcoholic. His parents were both alcoholics, as well. The patient tearfully asks the nurse whether this is a genetic condition, and what are the chances her child will have a problem with alcohol abuse.

    a. What other assessments should the nurse make?

    b. How should the nurse answer the patient's questions?

    c. What other interventions might the nurse include in the care plan for helping the patient deal with this situation?

27. A 50-year-old man has been admitted to the hospital with a diagnosis of advanced hypertension. He informs the nurse that he quit taking his medications several weeks ago. During the initial assessment, the nurse determines that the patient has excellent prescription drug insurance coverage.

    a. What other factors related to use of his medications must be assessed in this situation?

    b. The nurse determines that the patient has little knowledge regarding his medications and plans patient teaching as one of the primary nursing interventions. What information does the nurse need to give the patient regarding the use of his antihypertensives?

28. A woman has been admitted to the nurse's floor with multiple compression fractures of her lumbar vertebrae. On the nurse's initial assessment, the patient is obviously in pain—her face is pale, diaphoretic, and drawn. She is gripping the side rail with her hand. When the nurse offers her a narcotic for pain relief she refuses, saying, "It's not God's will for us to use medicines that cloud the mind so that we can't think about His goodness to us."

    a. What other modes of treatment could the nurse include in the care plan that the patient might find more compatible with her religious beliefs?

    b. What other assessments should the nurse make on the patient in order to help her further?

    c. Are there any medications the patient might be willing to consider if the nurse offered them?

CHAPTER 10

HERBAL AND ALTERNATIVE THERAPIES

FILL IN THE BLANK

From the textbook, find the correct word(s) to complete the statement(s).

1. Many people think the advantage of natural substances is that they have more _____ _____ than traditional drugs.

2. From the perspective of pharmacology, the value of complementary and alternative medicine (CAM) therapies lies in their ability to _____ the need for _____.

3. The nurse should not be _____ when the patient requests alternative treatment.

4. An herb is technically a botanical without any _____ _____.

5. When using herbs, it is essential to know which portion of the plant contains the _____ _____.

6. Herbal products are regulated by the _____ _____ _____ _____ _____ Act.

Adams/Holland, *Student Workbook and Resource Guide for Pharmacology for Nurses* 4th Edition
© 2014 by Pearson Education, Inc.

MATCHING

For questions 7 through 16, match the example in column I with the therapy name in column II.

Column I	Column II
7. _____ faith and prayer	a. biologic-based therapy
8. _____ yoga	b. alternate health care system
9. _____ biofeedback	c. manual healing
10. _____ nutritional supplements	d. mind-body intervention
11. _____ homeopathy	e. spiritual
12. _____ acupuncture, Chinese herbs	
13. _____ chiropractic	
14. _____ music, dance	
15. _____ shamans	
16. _____ massage	

MULTIPLE CHOICE

17. Common characteristics of CAM systems include all of the following EXCEPT:

    a. they consider the health of the whole person.

    b. they promote disease prevention, self-care, and self-healing.

    c. they recognize the role of spirituality in health and healing.

    d. they provide inexpensive supplements and substitutes for expensive traditional drugs.

18. Why did interest in herbal medicine begin to wane when the pharmaceutical industry rose in popularity in the late 1800s?

    a. Herbs became very expensive.

    b. Herbs were no longer readily available in the environment.

    c. Synthetic drugs could be standardized and produced more cheaply.

    d. Herbs were proved to be ineffective against most diseases.

19. Which of the following is NOT a major factor contributing to the steady increase in popularity of herbal products?

    a. Many herbs have been demonstrated to be more effective than available drugs.

    b. Herbal products are more widely available to the public.

    c. The herbal industry has aggressively marketed its products.

    d. Herbal products cost considerably less than most prescription medicines.

20. The nurse should understand that which of the following statements regarding herbs is false?

    a. Herbs may contain dozens of active chemicals.

    b. The chemicals in herbs may not have the same activity if they are isolated from each other.

c. Herbal supplements are standardized and the exact quantities of active ingredients are known.

d. The strength of an herbal preparation may vary depending on where it was grown and how it was stored.

21. Products intended to enhance the diet such as botanicals, vitamins, minerals, or any other extract or metabolite that is not already approved as a drug by the FDA are defined as which of the following?

a. Herbal products

b. Alternative therapies

c. Supplemental therapies

d. Dietary supplements

22. Which of the following is a legal requirement contained in the Dietary Supplement Health and Education Act (DSHEA)?

a. Dietary supplements must be tested for safety prior to marketing.

b. Effectiveness must be demonstrated by the manufacturer.

c. The herbal product must contain only one active ingredient.

d. Dietary supplements must state that the product is not intended to diagnose, treat, cure, or prevent any disease.

23. The nurse is teaching a patient about how to properly read labels on herbal products. The nurse should explain that which of the following statements would most likely NOT be allowed on the label of a dietary supplement?

a. Helps promote a healthy immune system

b. May reduce pain and inflammation

c. May reduce blood pressure and the risk of stroke

d. May improve cardiovascular function

24. The nurse is advising the patient about the proper use of herbal and dietary supplements. What is the responsibility of the nurse in regard to recommending herbal products?

a. Seek to dissuade the patient from using them because they are not "scientific."

b. Be aware of the latest medical information on herbal products including interactions and side effects.

c. Inform patients that they can trust the labeling on herbal products because the U.S. government has a rigorous testing program before the product is marketed.

d. Tell the patient to seek information on herbal products from a practitioner of alternative medicine rather than a physician, because most physicians have no knowledge of these products.

25. The nurse should know that which popular herb is used for its possible benefit in treating depression?

a. Aloe

b. Bilberry

c. St. John's wort

d. Ginger

26. The patient has asked the nurse which herb may have beneficial effects on the immune system. The nurse should know that which of the following popular herbs is used for this purpose?

a. Black cohosh

b. Echinacea

c. Ginkgo

d. Evening primrose

27. While assessing a new patient, the nurse discovers that he is taking saw palmetto daily. The nurse should know that this popular herb is taken for what potential effect?

    a. Relief of urinary problems related to enlarged prostate

    b. Reduction of stress and to promote sleep

    c. Reduction of blood cholesterol levels

    d. Treatment of constipation

28. A female patient with insulin-dependent diabetes presents with complaints of frequent hypoglycemic episodes. She tells the nurse that she is taking all of the following dietary supplements. Which one may be contributing to her hypoglycemia?

    a. Ginger

    b. Ginkgo biloba

    c. Echinacea

    d. Garlic

29. The Dietary Supplement and Nonprescription Drug Consumer Protection Act requires the companies marketing herbal and dietary supplements to:

    a. prove the effectiveness of the product prior to marketing.

    b. ensure the safety of the product in children and older adults.

    c. include contact information on the product labels for consumers to use in reporting adverse events.

    d. provide comprehensive safety information to the consumer on their websites.

MAKING CONNECTIONS

30. Which of the following choices distinguishes a conventional drug from a natural alternative agent?

    a. A natural alternative agent is obtained from a natural source.

    b. A conventional drug is routinely prescribed by health care providers.

    c. A conventional drug is synthetically produced.

    d. A natural alternative must be tested by the FDA.

31. Which of the following statements best describes an advantage of prescription drugs over OTC drugs?

    a. OTC drugs do not require a physician's order.

    b. Prescription drugs ensure that harmful reactions will not occur.

    c. When prescribed by their health care provider, patients will take only prescription medications.

    d. The health care provider can maximize therapy by ordering the amount and frequency to be dispensed.

32. The nurse reads an order for chlorpromazine 50 mg every 6 h PR. Which of the following is a rationale for administering a drug by the rectal route to a patient?

    a. The patient is unconscious.

    b. The patient is experiencing nausea or vomiting.

    c. The patient is an infant who cannot swallow pills.

    d. All of the above are correct.

33. The nurse should understand that which of the following drug administration methods should be used when rapid results are required?

    a. Intravenous

    b. Intramuscular

    c. Oral

    d. Rectal

34. The patient who is most likely to benefit from a prescription drug is the one who:

    a. has prescription drug coverage through an insurance company.

    b. sees the physician regularly and follows the directions for using the drug.

    c. is not aware that the drug can cause serious adverse effects.

    d. uses herbal supplements and goes to the health care provider when these fail to work.

CASE STUDY APPLICATIONS

35. A 78-year-old man is being discharged from the nurse's unit on digoxin (Lanoxin) and warfarin (Coumadin). The care plan includes patient education regarding these drugs. The nurse has included the patient's wife in the teaching session, and she mentions that she believes his problems can be corrected by using herbs rather than drugs. The patient states, "I'm going to do what the doctor says, but a few weeds can't hurt me. I'll take them to keep her happy."

    a. What further assessments are indicated in this situation?

    b. The care plan has been altered to give additional information on herbal preparations to this couple. What information must the nurse give to the patient and his wife regarding the use of herbs while on Coumadin and Lanoxin?

    c. What other information regarding the use of herbal products should be given to this patient?

36. A woman comes to the mental health outpatient clinic with new symptoms, including agitation, headache, and dizziness. The nurse notes on assessment that the patient is also profusely diaphoretic. The patient has been treated for depression with Prozac, a selective serotonin reuptake inhibitor (SSRI). During the nurse's assessment, the patient confides that she has been using St. John's wort with her prescription drugs. She asks if her prescription can be changed to something that "works better."

    a. What is a possible cause of the patient's symptoms?

    b. The nurse's initial plan of care is for patient education regarding drug–herb interactions. What other antidepressants might interact unfavorably with St. John's wort?

37. A 42-year-old man has been using echinacea regularly, yet he now has the flu. The nurse notes during the assessment that the patient has rheumatoid arthritis, for which he is taking methotrexate. The patient is upset that he has become ill and feels that the advertisements in nutrition magazines and on television may have misled him into buying useless products. He asks for the nurse's advice regarding the value of alternative therapies.

    a. The nursing interventions call for monitoring specific lab values in view of the patient's use of echinacea and methotrexate. Using a Drug Guide, which lab values would the nurse monitor, and why?

    b. The care plan includes patient education regarding the uses of alternative therapies. What information should be included?

    c. During team conference, a colleague suggests that a goal for the patient's care should be "discontinues use of all supplements and uses only prescription drugs." Describe why the nurse disagrees with the colleague's suggestion, and write an improved goal.

CHAPTER 11

SUBSTANCE ABUSE

FILL IN THE BLANK

From the textbook, find the correct word(s) to complete the statement(s).

1. The most commonly abused drugs are _____ and _____.

2. Three substances that come from natural sources and are frequently abused are _____, _____, and _____.

3. _____ is a biologic condition that occurs when the body adapts to a substance after repeated administration; when this condition extends to closely related drugs it is called _____ _____.

4. Two categories used to classify substance dependence are _____ _____ and _____ _____.

5. _____ is an overwhelming compulsion that drives someone to take drugs repetitively, despite serious health and social consequences.

6. Psychological dependence may develop after one dose of _____ _____.

7. It is common to treat alcohol withdrawal with a short-acting _____.

8. Drugs used in the treatment of opioid dependence include _____, _____, and _____.

9. After several months of pain therapy, a patient must increase the dose of the pain medication. The best description of this situation is that the patient has developed _____ to the pain medication.

10. Signs of physical discomfort after drug use is discontinued are referred to as classic _____ _____.

Adams/Holland, *Student Workbook and Resource Guide for Pharmacology for Nurses* 4th Edition
© 2014 by Pearson Education, Inc.

MATCHING

For questions 11 through 18, match the drug or substance in column I with its group name in column II.

Column I	Column II
11. _____ lysergic acid diethylamide (LSD)	a. hallucinogen
12. _____ nicotine	b. CNS stimulant
13. _____ alprazolam (Xanax)	c. CNS depressant
14. _____ oxycodone (OxyContin)	d. opioid
15. _____ dextroamphetamine (Dexedrine)	
16. _____ methylphenidate (Ritalin)	
17. _____ hydrocodone and acetaminophen combination (Vicodin)	
18. _____ MDMA (Ecstasy)	

For questions 19 through 23, match the characteristic signs of toxicity in column I with their drug classification in column II.

Column I	Column II
19. _____ somnolence	a. opioid
20. _____ diminished reflexes	b. nicotine
21. _____ cyanosis	c. cocaine
22. _____ heart palpitations	d. benzodiazepine
23. _____ dysrhythmias	e. alcohol

For questions 24 through 27, match the drug/substance in column I with its source in column II.

Column I	Column II
24. _____ opium	a. natural
25. _____ mescaline	b. synthetic
26. _____ cocaine	
27. _____ LSD	

MULTIPLE CHOICE

28. All abused substances affect which body system?

    a. Cardiovascular

    b. Nervous

    c. Digestive

    d. Respiratory

29. The nurse is working with a patient who has a diagnosis of alcoholism. What organ system is most likely to be malfunctioning for this patient?

    a. Lungs

    b. Bowels

    c. Liver

    d. Kidneys

30. A patient is admitted with liver failure. What nursing action is most appropriate prior to delivery of medications for this patient?

    a. Check drug dosing because of issues related to metabolism.

    b. Request increase in blood clotting drugs because of liver dysfunction.

    c. Hold all nutritional supplements until liver disease is resolved.

    d. Expect increase in drug dosing of antibiotics because of immune compromise.

31. Repeated use of caffeine products can create which of the following effects?

    a. Decreased stomach acid

    b. Decreased blood pressure

    c. Increased fatigue

    d. Increased urination

32. What drug was once used for bronchodilation but has been discontinued because of psychotic episodes in some patients?

    a. Cocaine

    b. LSD

    c. Phencyclidine

    d. Amphetamine

33. Which of the following statements about addiction is NOT correct?

    a. Addiction is most likely a neurobiologic problem linked closely to the patient's psychological state and social setting.

    b. In some cases, addiction may begin with the patient's medical need for the treatment of an illness.

    c. The therapeutic use of narcotics and sedatives creates large numbers of addicted patients.

    d. Attempts to predict a patient's addictive tendency using psychological profiles or genetic markers have largely been unsuccessful.

34. Which of the following drugs was once used as a local anesthetic?

    a. Amphetamine

    b. Ketamine

    c. Phencyclidine

    d. Cocaine

35. Irritability, restlessness, insomnia, tremor, chills, and weight loss are characteristic withdrawal symptoms of:

    a. marijuana

    b. nicotine

    c. opioids

    d. hallucinogens

36. Which of the following statements about tolerance is *not* correct?

    a. Patients often endure annoying side effects if they know that tolerance to these effects will develop quickly.

    b. Tolerance to mood-altering drugs and their ability to reduce pain develops more slowly.

    c. Tolerance never develops to the drug's ability to constrict the pupils.

    d. Patients develop tolerance to the nausea and vomiting produced by narcotics only after multiple doses.

37. For which sleep disorder drug class do patients often try to fake or modify prescriptions?

    a. Amphetamines

    b. Barbiturates

    c. Benzodiazepines

    d. Opioids

CASE STUDY APPLICATIONS

38. A 28-year-old patient is admitted to the hospital with pneumonia. During the nurse's assessment of the social history, the nurse learns that the patient has a job, is self-reliant, and smokes marijuana every other night, but does not drink alcohol. The patient claims "smoking a joint now and then doesn't hurt anybody."

    a. What would the nurse teach this patient regarding the long-term effects of marijuana?

    b. Describe the psychological effects of marijuana and explain how dependence might develop in this case.

    c. Compare the marijuana risks to those of smoking tobacco products.

39. A patient admitted for recurrent bladder infections describes a 15-year history of drinking beer and wine in moderate amounts. The patient gives a family history of paternal alcoholism. The patient asks, "What kinds of factors are linked with addiction? Is it genetic, or is there some other reason why people become addicted?"

    a. What would the nurse include in the teaching plan to answer the patient's questions?

    b. What assessment data are important when the nurse admits this patient?

    c. What nursing diagnoses and patient outcomes are appropriate for this patient?

CHAPTER 12

EMERGENCY PREPAREDNESS AND POISONINGS

FILL IN THE BLANK

From the textbook, find the correct word(s) to complete the statement(s).

1. Traditional infectious diseases include possible epidemics caused by _____, _____, _____, and _____.

2. The program designed to supply essential medical equipment to a community in the event of a disaster is called _____ _____ _____.

3. _____ _____ are fully stocked sets of preassembled supplies that can be sent to a community in the United States within 12 hours after a bioterrorist attack.

4. The anthrax vaccine causes the body to make _____ _____ that prevent the onset of disease.

5. Nerve agent antidote injector kits contain the anticholinergic drug _____.

6. Potassium iodide is effective in preventing radiation-induced thyroid cancer even if taken _____ hours after radiation exposure.

Adams/Holland, *Student Workbook and Resource Guide for Pharmacology for Nurses* 4th Edition
© 2014 by Pearson Education, Inc.

MATCHING

For questions 7 through 13, match the information in column I with its disease in column II.

Column I

7. _____ found in contaminated animal products such as wool, hair, bonemeal

8. _____ oral vaccine available

9. _____ caused by variola virus

10. _____ genetic code is public information

11. _____ ciprofloxacin used for prophylaxis

12. _____ can be manufactured in a simple laboratory

13. _____ could cause mortality in as many as one in three persons if released into unvaccinated population

Column II

a. anthrax

b. smallpox

c. polio

For questions 14 through 21, match the chemical agent in column II with the treatment in column I.

Column I

14. _____ atropine

15. _____ give milk to drink

16. _____ sodium thiosulfate 1% to induce emesis

17. _____ fresh air and oxygen

18. _____ rinse nose and throat with 10% solution of sodium bicarbonate

19. _____ treat skin with borated talcum powder

20. _____ treat skin with 10% solution of sodium carbonate

21. _____ oxygen and amyl nitrate

Column II

a. nerve agents (sarin, soman, tabun)

b. lewisite

c. phosgene (gas)

d. hydrogen cyanide

e. adamsite-DM

Adams/Holland, *Student Workbook and Resource Guide for Pharmacology for Nurses* 4th Edition
© 2014 by Pearson Education, Inc.

For questions 22 through 30, match the overdosed substance or toxin in column II with the specific antidote in column I.

Column I	Column II
22. _____ digitoxin	a. acetylcysteine
23. _____ lead toxicity	b. calcium EDTA
24. _____ benzodiazepine overdose	c. digoxin immune Fab
25. _____ iron toxicity	d. dimercaprol
26. _____ methotrexate	e. deferoxamine
27. _____ mercury toxicity	f. flumazenil
28. _____ neuromuscular blocking agents	g. leucovorin
29. _____ radioactive plutonium	h. neostigmine
30. _____ acetaminophen	i. penetrate zinc trisodium

MULTIPLE CHOICE

31. Which of these is NOT an area of concern for possible use by bioterrorists?

    a. Infectious diseases such as anthrax and plague

    b. Incapacitating chemicals such as nerve gas and cyanide

    c. Common drugs such as morphine and strong antibiotics

    d. Nuclear and radiation exposures

32. When do the symptoms of anthrax exposure usually appear?

    a. 1 to 6 days after exposure

    b. 2 to 10 days after exposure

    c. 12 to 24 hours after exposure

    d. 1 week to 1 month after exposure

33. The public is discouraged from using antibiotics prophylactically unless there is a confirmed exposure to anthrax. All of the following are rationales for this policy EXCEPT:

    a. unnecessary use of antibiotics can be expensive.

    b. antibiotics can cause significant side effects.

    c. unnecessary use of antibiotics promotes the development of resistant bacteria.

    d. antibiotic use may inactivate the anthrax vaccine.

34. The smallpox vaccine is contraindicated for all of the following persons EXCEPT:

    a. a 25-year-old who is HIV positive.

    b. an individual who has already been exposed to the disease.

    c. a nursing mother.

    d. an individual with eczema.

35. Exposure to any of the nerve agents can cause all of the following symptoms EXCEPT:

    a. respiratory failure and convulsions.

    b. severe nausea and vomiting.

    c. increased sweating and salivation.

    d. incontinence of urine and stool.

36. Radiation sickness is also known as which of the following?

    a. Acute radiation exposure

    b. Acute radiation syndrome

    c. Nuclear exposure syndrome

    d. Radioisotope syndrome

37. Which of the effects of radiation exposure may be prevented if potassium iodide is used within 3 to 4 hours of exposure to ionizing radiation?

    a. Leukemia

    b. Nausea, vomiting, diarrhea

    c. Thyroid cancer

    d. Bone marrow suppression

38. Recent Joint Commission standards for emergency management include all of the following EXCEPT:

    a. response to immediate casualties.

    b. how an agency's health care delivery will change during a crisis.

    c. disposition of fatalities.

    d. coordination of agencies' efforts with community resources.

39. Which of the following statements regarding the role of the nurse in emergency preparedness is NOT correct?

    a. The nurse must maintain current knowledge of emergency management related to bioterrorist activities.

    b. The nurse must be aware of the early signs and symptoms of chemical and biologic agents, and their immediate treatment.

    c. The nurse should be involved in developing emergency plans.

    d. The nurse should prepare for bioterrorist activities by receiving all available vaccines against biologic agents.

40. *Bacillus anthracis* can be transmitted in all of the following ways EXCEPT:

    a. bite by an insect that carries the disease.

    b. exposure through an open wound.

    c. contaminated food.

    d. inhalation.

CASE STUDY APPLICATIONS

41. During a routine visit to her health care provider, the patient confides to the nurse that she is "terrified" of getting anthrax, even though no new cases have been reported in quite some time. She wants a supply of drugs to prevent an infection. The nurse notes that she becomes agitated while discussing terrorism, wringing her hands and looking distressed. The nursing diagnosis is "*Deficient Knowledge* related to bioterrorism/anthrax as evidenced by questions voiced and nonverbal anxiety behaviors."

    a. The care plan includes interventions relating to patient education. What information would the nurse give the patient regarding prophylactic use of antibiotics for bioterrorism agents?

    b. What information would the nurse give the patient about the anthrax vaccine?

42. The nurse is asked to assist in the writing of a protocol for the administration of smallpox vaccine to health care workers and law enforcement personnel in the local area.

    a. What nursing assessments would be included prior to the administration of the vaccine?

    b. What information should be included in a pamphlet handed to each person who plans to be vaccinated?

43. A man who lives within 2 miles of a nuclear power plant comes to the health care provider's office to request "the pills that make you immune to radiation sickness." Because the nurse is aware that nurses play a key role in educating the public regarding bioterrorism, the nurse has developed a standard care plan regarding nuclear disaster education for patients who live near the power plant.

    a. What patient teaching should the nurse give to the patient regarding potassium iodide?

    b. In evaluating the patient's understanding of the information he has been given, the nurse asks him to explain why potassium iodide is effective in preventing thyroid cancer after radiation exposure. What answer would be correct?

CHAPTER 13

DRUGS AFFECTING THE AUTONOMIC NERVOUS SYSTEM

FILL IN THE BLANK

From the textbook, find the correct word(s) to complete the statement(s).

1. The two primary divisions of the nervous system are the _____ nervous system, composed of the brain and spinal cord, and the _____ nervous system, composed of sensory and motor pathways.

2. The _____ nervous system provides involuntary control over smooth muscle, cardiac muscle, and glands.

3. The sympathetic nervous system produces the _____ response; the parasympathetic nervous system produces symptoms called the _____ response.

4. _____ is the main neurotransmitter responsible for sympathetic nervous transmission; _____ is the main neurotransmitter responsible for parasympathetic nervous transmission.

5. Sympathetic nerves are often called _____, a term coming from the word *adrenaline*; parasympathetic nerves are called _____.

6. Increased heart rate, bronchodilation, decreased motility in the GI tract, mydriasis, and decreased secretions from glands are physiologic responses associated with inactivation of the _____ nervous system or activation of the _____ nervous system coming from the word *acetylcholine*.

7. _____ _____, primarily used for hypertension, produce actions *opposite* those of the sympathomimetics.

8. A class of drugs named after the fight-or-flight response and primarily used for increasing the heart rate, dilating the bronchi, and drying secretions resulting from colds is _____ drugs.

9. _____ drugs, named after the rest-and-digest response, are commonly used to stimulate the urinary or digestive tracts following general anesthesia.

Adams/Holland, *Student Workbook and Resource Guide for Pharmacology for Nurses* 4th Edition
© 2014 by Pearson Education, Inc.

MATCHING

For questions 10 through 14, match the physiologic responses in column I with the autonomic receptor classes in column II.

Column I

10. _____ cause dry mouth, constipation, urinary retention, and increased heart rate

11. _____ relax vascular smooth muscle and dry nasal secretions

12. _____ cause bronchodilation

13. _____ lower blood pressure without affecting the heart

14. _____ decrease heart rate

Column II

a. beta$_1$ blockers

b. alpha$_1$ blockers

c. beta$_2$ agonists

d. alpha$_2$ agonists

e. cholinergic (muscarinic) blockers

For questions 15 through 19, match the peripheral nervous system drug in column I with the indication in column II.

Column I

15. _____ atropine (Atropen)

16. _____ bethanechol (Duvoid, Urecholine)

17. _____ pyridostigmine (Mestinon, Regonol)

18. _____ doxazosin (Cardura)

19. _____ albuterol (Proventil, Ventolin, VoSpire)

Column II

a. myasthenia gravis

b. GI stimulation following surgery

c. poisoning with anticholinesterase agents

d. asthma inhaler

e. hypertension

For questions 20 through 24, match the drug in column I with the classification in column II.

Column I

20. _____ scopolamine (Hyoscine, Transderm-Scop)

21. _____ phenylephrine (Neo-Synephrine)

22. _____ bethanechol (Duvoid, Urecholine)

23. _____ propranolol (Inderal, Innopran XL)

24. _____ dobutamine (Dobutrex)

Column II

a. parasympathomimetic

b. anticholinergic

c. sympathomimetic

d. adrenergic blocker (antagonist)

MULTIPLE CHOICE

25. A patient is discharged with a newly prescribed antagonist for control of hypertension. The nurse gives discharge instructions. Which of the following discharge instructions is inappropriate?

   a. Report any difficulty with urination to the nurse.

   b. Take the medication for the first time directly prior to getting into bed.

   c. Monitor blood pressure and pulse daily, giving parameters that need to be reported.

   d. Return for lab tests to monitor renal function.

26. An cholinergic blocker is most directly related to which of the following?

   a. Stimulation of the sympathetic nervous system

   b. Inhibition of the parasympathetic nervous system

   c. Stimulation of the parasympathetic nervous system

   d. Inhibition of the sympathetic nervous system

27. How does bethanechol (Duvoid, Urecholine) exert its effects?

   a. Stimulates cholinergic receptors

   b. Blocks cholinergic receptors

   c. Blocks beta receptors

   d. Stimulates alpha receptors

28. What drugs block the action of norepinephrine at alpha and beta receptors?

   a. Parasympathomimetics

   b. Parasympatholytics

   c. Sympathomimetics

   d. Sympatholytics

29. A nurse is to give phenylephrine parenterally. What safety precaution would be necessary, especially with this drug?

   a. Monitor patency throughout the infusion.

   b. Monitor patient's temperature every 1 hour during the infusion.

   c. Monitor for CNS depression.

   d. Monitor for hypotension throughout the infusion.

30. Parasympathomimetics are safe for patients diagnosed with which of the following?

   a. Myasthenia gravis

   b. GI obstruction

   c. Asthma

   d. Angina or dysrhythmias

31. How does propranolol (Inderal, Innopran XL) exert its effects?

    a. Stimulates cholinergic receptors

    b. Blocks cholinergic receptors

    c. Blocks beta receptors

    d. Stimulates alpha receptors

32. Pseudoephedrine has been ordered for a patient with nasal congestion. The nurse knows the drug can give which of the following side effects?

    a. Hypertension, insomnia, and tachycardia

    b. Drowsiness and dry mouth

    c. Increased heart rate and abdominal cramps

    d. Dilated pupils and orthostatic hypotension

33. An anticholinergic may be used in treatment of peptic ulcers. What action makes this drug useful in this condition?

    a. Decreases gastric emptying time

    b. Decreases gastric acid secretions

    c. Decreases intestinal motility

    d. Relaxes gastric smooth muscles

34. What are sympathomimetics also called?

    a. Cholinergic agonists

    b. Adrenergic agonists

    c. Cholinergic blockers

    d. Adrenergic blockers

35. Epinephrine is a nonselective adrenergic agonist. What is the disadvantage of this nonspecific action?

    a. It causes more autonomic side effects.

    b. This drug cannot be used for nervous system conditions.

    c. It will not cross the blood–brain barrier.

    d. It can only be given by SC injection.

36. A patient is prescribed pyridostigmine (Mestinon, Regonol) for myasthenia gravis. Which of the following would be inappropriate to teach the patient?

    a. Take the drug at the same times each day.

    b. Take drug on a full stomach.

    c. Monitor liver enzymes as requested.

    d. Maintain a journal of episodes of weakness and how long after drug administration they occur.

37. Neostigmine (Prostigmin) is an example of which of the following?

    a. Cholinergic blocker

    b. Nicotinic blocker

    c. Cholinergic agonist

    d. Cholinesterase inhibitor

38. Which of the following drugs would dry up body secretions?

    a. Bethanechol (Duvoid, Urecholine)

    b. Metoprolol (Lopressor, Toprol)

    c. Atropine (AtroPen)

    d. Doxazosin (Cardura)

39. Atropine is usually not prescribed for any patient with glaucoma. The nurse knows the contraindication is due to which of the following effects of atropine?

    a. Increases intraocular pressure

    b. Decreases lacrimation

    c. Decreases lateral movement of the eyes

    d. Increases difficulty with night vision due to papillary constriction

MAKING CONNECTIONS

40. Methylphenidate (Ritalin) is most similar to which abused substance?

    a. Tetrahydrocannabinol (THC)

    b. Ketamine

    c. Methamphetamine

    d. Ethyl alcohol

41. When a drug is referred to as an agonist, it can do which of the following?

    a. Be a facilitator of an action

    b. Be an inhibitor of an action

    c. Have a potentiated action

    d. Make one drug interact with another drug

42. What is (are) the most commonly abused sympathomimetic(s)?

    a. Amphetamines

    b. Proventil

    c. Sudafed/pseudoephedrine

    d. Marijuana

43. What is an example of an illegal CNS stimulant?

    a. Propoxyphene (Darvon)

    b. Flurazepam (Dalmane)

    c. Heroin

    d. Cocaine

44. The nurse is to administer medications using the "five rights." Giving medications to a patient without an ID bracelet violates which of the rights?

    a. Right medications

    b. Right time

    c. Right patient

    d. Right route

CALCULATIONS

45. The physician orders metaproterenol sulfate 20 mg four times a day. The pharmacy sends metaproterenol syrup 10 mg/5 cc. The patient should receive _____ cc per day.

46. The physician orders 0.3 mg atropine sulfate SC every 4 h. The pharmacy sends atropine sulfate 0.6 mg/mL. The nurse should administer _____ mL SC every 4 h.

CASE STUDY APPLICATIONS

47. An 80-year-old male patient has been diagnosed with COPD and hypertension. The patient has been given propranolol (Inderal) to treat the hypertension. The nurse is assessing the following medications that he is also taking: Benadryl 25 mg every 4 h for itching and sneezing due to allergies, Prazosin bid for hypertension, and Proventil inhaler prn for wheezing.

    a. Identify three potential nursing diagnoses that could occur because of drug interactions when these medications are given concurrently. Explain why these interactions would occur.

    b. What nursing interventions can be done to decrease the risk of the problems created with these interactions?

48. A female patient diagnosed with myasthenia gravis comes to the emergency department with muscle weakness. The nurse, during the history, determines that the patient has been taking double doses of pyridostigmine (Mestinon) over the past several days.

    a. What assessment would the nurse make to identify a nursing diagnosis?

    b. What nursing diagnosis would the nurse identify?

    c. What nursing interventions could be used in this diagnosis?

CHAPTER 14

DRUGS FOR ANXIETY AND INSOMNIA

FILL IN THE BLANK

From the textbook, find the correct word(s) to complete the statement(s).

1. Apprehension, tension, or uneasiness lasting for 6 months or longer and causing considerable stress is referred to as _____ _____ _____.

2. Two important sets of brain structures are associated with anxiety. One connected with emotion is the _____ system; the other, projecting from the brainstem and connected with alertness, is the _____ _____ system.

3. _____ are classes of drugs prescribed to relax patients. Classes of drugs used to help patients to sleep are _____.

4. Diazepam (Valium) reduces anxiety by binding to a receptor in the brain referred to as the _____ _____ – _____ channel molecule.

5. The drug class usually prescribed for short-term insomnia caused by anxiety is _____.

6. _____ is a class of drugs that reduces anxiety, causes drowsiness, and promotes sleep when administered at higher doses.

7. _____ _____ is a fatal symptom often associated with an overdose of barbiturates and other CNS depressants.

8. Schedule _____ is the level assigned to many benzodiazepines; Schedule _____ is the level assigned to some barbiturates.

9. _____ have an ability to reduce anxiety symptoms by altering levels of norepinephrine, dopamine, and/or serotonin in the brain.

Adams/Holland, *Student Workbook and Resource Guide for Pharmacology for Nurses* 4th Edition
© 2014 by Pearson Education, Inc.

MATCHING

For questions 10 through 14, match the descriptions in column I with its drug classification in column II.

Column I

10. _____ beginning in the early 1900s, the drug classification used to control seizures, insomnia, and anxiety

11. _____ class containing drugs that act by binding GABA, intensifying the effect, without causing respiratory depression unless taken with other CNS depressants

12. _____ reduce anxiety symptoms but are chemically different from the other main anxiolytic drug classes.

13. _____ class of drugs that have an FDA black box to warn patients of potentially harmful effects

14. _____ a chemical related to tryptophan, sold OTC

Column II

a. benzodiazepines

b. barbiturates

c. nonbenzodiazepines, nonbarbiturate sedatives

d. melatonin

e. antidepressants

For questions 15 through 20, match the drug in column I with its class name and most appropriate use in column II.

Column I

15. _____ secobarbital (Seconal)

16. _____ escitalopram (Lexapro)

17. _____ zolpidem (Ambien)

18. _____ lorazepam (Ativan)

19. _____ amobarbital (Amytal)

20. _____ zaleplon (Sonata)

Column II

a. benzodiazepine for anxiety and panic

b. benzodiazepine for short-term relief of insomnia

c. intermediate-acting barbiturate with sedative and hypnotic properties for short-term relief of insomnia

d. short-acting barbiturate with sedative and hypnotic properties

e. nonbarbiturate CNS depressant for short-term relief of insomnia

f. antidepressant indicated for generalized anxiety disorder; unlabeled use for treatment of panic disorders

MULTIPLE CHOICE

21. What term describes episodes of immediate and intense apprehension, fearfulness, or terror?

    a. Anxiety

    b. Panic

    c. Phobia

    d. Post-traumatic stress

22. What drug category should be avoided for patients receiving MAOI therapy?

    a. Anxiolytics

    b. Sedatives

    c. Mood disorder drugs

    d. Antidepressants

23. Benzodiazepines have several uses. Which use would NOT be appropriate?

    a. Long-term administration to treat phobias, OCD, and PTSD

    b. When anxiety interferes with daily activities of living

    c. Short-term treatment of generalized anxiety disorder

    d. Short-term treatment of insomnia caused by anxiety

24. Which of the following terms may be used to describe benzodiazepines?

    a. Sedative

    b. Hypnotic

    c. Tranquilizer

    d. All of the above

25. What was one of the first drugs used for anxiety treatment?

    a. Alprazolam (Xanax)

    b. Clonazepam (Klonopin)

    c. Chlordiazepoxide (Librium)

    d. Clorazepate (Tranxene)

26. CNS depressants include which of the following drug classes?

    a. Benzodiazepines

    b. Barbiturates

    c. Nonbarbiturates, nonbenzodiazepine sedatives

    d. All of the above

27. Which statement is true about re-establishing a healthful sleep regimen?

    a. Drinking alcohol close to bedtime helps one to sleep.

    b. Eating a moderate meal close to bedtime helps one to sleep.

    c. Supplements are often recommended for insomnia.

    d. Sedatives and hypnotics may be useful for insomnia if taken long term.

28. Which of the following best describes rebound insomnia?

    a. A time during which insomnia and symptoms of anxiety may worsen

    b. A worsening of insomnia due to drug dependency

    c. More common in younger patients

    d. Develops from short-term use of insomnia medication

29. Melatonin can be bought OTC for insomnia. Which patient teaching would be appropriate for this supplement?

    a. Melatonin can increase ovulation in women trying to conceive.

    b. Melatonin can be taken safely during pregnancy.

    c. Melatonin can safely be given to patients who are on steroids.

    d. Melatonin is not regulated by the FDA, but sold OTC without a prescription.

30. Which of the following is true regarding sleep stages and patterns?

    a. Drugs for insomnia generally do not affect sleep stages.

    b. Patients with normal sleep patterns move from non-REM to REM sleep about every 90 minutes.

    c. REM sleep is the deepest stage of sleep.

    d. The most significant type of sleep with respect to the effect of hypnotic drugs is REM sleep.

31. Sleep deprivation has been linked to which of the following?

    a. Decreased risk of type 2 diabetes

    b. Becoming frightened, irritable, paranoid, and emotionally disturbed

    c. Less daydreaming or fantasizing throughout the day

    d. Better judgment and less impulsive thinking

32. Which of the following best describes phenobarbital?

    a. Is a short-acting barbiturate and thus more useful for brief medical procedures

    b. Stimulates liver enzymes and thus may increase its own metabolism with repeated dosing

    c. Is mainly limited in drug therapy for induction of sleep

    d. Does not affect levels of folate (B_9) or vitamin D in the body

33. Benzodiazepines must be given with caution when given parenterally because of what risk?

    a. Seizures

    b. CNS excitation

    c. Respiratory depression

    d. Dependence

34. Which of the following best describes buspirone (BuSpar)?

    a. Is a benzodiazepine

    b. May act by binding to brain dopamine and serotonin receptors

    c. Is used for short-term treatment of insomnia

    d. All of the above

MAKING CONNECTIONS

35. A patient is experiencing extreme anxiety in a dental chair due to an impending tooth extraction. Which route of administration should the dentist use to give the most rapid onset of action of a drug for anxiety?

    a. Oral

    b. IV

    c. IM

    d. Rectal

36. Scopolamine (Transderm-Scop) is an anticholinergic agent. Which of the following is least likely to be a side effect of this drug?

    a. Dry mouth

    b. Bradycardia

    c. Tachycardia

    d. Urinary retention

37. Which of the following drug delivery methods is NOT a parenteral method of drug delivery and thus avoids the first-pass effect in the liver?

    a. Oral

    b. Intrathecal

    c. Intramuscular

    d. Sublingual

38. One reason the first-pass effect is so important is that drugs absorbed at the level of the digestive tract do which of the following?

    a. Are circulated directly back to the heart

    b. Are distributed to the rest of the body and target organs

    c. Have ultimately more bioavailability than they would if absorbed at a different location

    d. Are routed through the hepatic portal circulation

39. Younger and elder patients metabolize drugs _____ than middle-age patients.

    a. More slowly

    b. More rapidly

    c. At the same rate

CALCULATIONS

40. A physician orders lorazepam 1.5 mg IV bolus. The pharmacy supplies 0.001 g/mL of lorazepam. The nurse should administer _____ mL IV bolus as ordered.

41. The physician orders diazepam 1 mg solution PO. The oral solution is 5 mg/mL. The nurse should administer _____ mL/dose.

CASE STUDY APPLICATIONS

42. A 38-year-old male patient is to have a short surgical procedure during which he will be given Versed IV. The nurse knows that Versed is a short-acting benzodiazepine.

   a. What does the nurse need to assess prior to giving Versed?

   b. What interventions would the nurse use to maintain the patient's safety during the procedure?

   c. What would the nurse use to evaluate the effectiveness of these interventions?

43. A female patient is troubled about a new job and has not slept in weeks. She feels that if she can just get through a couple more weeks, things might start to become a little easier. One thing that would definitely help her is a good night of sleep.

   a. What nursing diagnosis would the nurse identify for this patient?

   b. What nursing interventions would be used to assist this patient?

   c. What would the nurse teach the patient regarding available pharmacologic interventions?

CHAPTER 15

DRUGS FOR SEIZURES

FILL IN THE BLANK

From the textbook, find the correct word(s) to complete the statement(s).

1. A _____ is symptomatic of the disorder epilepsy, rather than being considered a disease in itself.

2. Six possible causes of seizures include _____, _____, _____
   _____, _____ _____, _____ _____, and
   _____ _____.

3. Because antiseizure drugs are mostly pregnancy category D, patients should use _____
   _____.

4. Antiseizure drugs may cause _____ deficiency, which can cause neural tube defects in a fetus.

5. Patients who have seizures may have a lower tolerance to environmental triggers such as _____
   deprivation and exposure to _____ or _____ lights.

6. _____ seizures occur in 0.5% of _____-month-old to _____-year-old
   children during an illness and last 1 to 2 minutes. Prevention is best carried out by controlling
   _____.

7. Of the major antiseizure medications, _____ is a drug of choice for a broader range of seizure
   types.

8. _____ seizures occur only on one side of the brain and continue for a short distance before they
   stop; _____ seizures may travel throughout the brain.

Adams/Holland, *Student Workbook and Resource Guide for Pharmacology for Nurses* 4th Edition
© 2014 by Pearson Education, Inc.

9. Of the most popular antiseizure medications, the drug of choice for absence seizures is _____.

10. Two popular medications used to treat status epilepticus are _____ and _____.

11. _____ _____ is an emergency type of generalized tonic-clonic seizure that is prolonged and usually affects _____, causing hypoxia.

12. Treatment of status epilepticus includes maintenance of the _____ and IV antiseizure medications.

13. The goal of antiseizure medications is to prevent _____ or repeated firing and therefore to _____ neuronal activity.

14. Once seizures are controlled, drug therapy continues for some time. After _____ years, the medications may be withdrawn slowly, one at a time, over several _____.

MATCHING

For questions 15 through 21, match the signs and symptoms in column I with its type of seizure in column II.

Column I

15. _____ In adults, this seizure may be preceded by an aura. Muscles then become tense, and a rhythmic jerking motion develops.

16. _____ This seizure is marked by major muscle groups contracting quickly, making a jerking motion. Patients appear unsteady and clumsy and may fall from a sitting position or drop whatever they are holding.

17. _____ This seizure usually starts with a blank stare. Patients may become disoriented and not pay attention to verbal commands or act as if they have a psychiatric illness. After the seizure, patients do not remember what happened.

18. _____ Patients may feel, for a brief moment, out of sorts and that their precise location is vague. Often, patients will hear and see things that are not there or may smell or taste things and have an upset stomach. Parts of the body such as the arms, legs, or face may start twitching. Symptoms are often not dramatic and may occur without loss of consciousness.

19. _____ This type of seizure occurs most often in children. Patients develop a blank stare without having twitching facial or body movements. This seizure lasts for only a few seconds. Patients then quickly recover and engage in normal activities.

Column II

a. simple partial seizure

b. complex partial seizure (psychomotor or temporal lobe seizure)

c. absence seizure (petit mal seizure)

d. atonic seizure (drop attack)

e. myoclonic seizure

f. generalized tonic-clonic seizure (grand mal seizure)

g. status epilepticus

20. _____ This is a medical emergency brought on by repeated seizures and convulsions. Steps must be taken to ensure that the airway remains open.

21. _____ Patients often stumble or fall for no apparent reason. Episodes are very short, lasting only a matter of seconds. After the seizure, patients return to normal activities without difficulty.

For questions 22 through 27, match the drug in column I with its pharmacologic category in Column II.

Column I	Column II
22. _____ acetazolamide (Diamox)	a. drugs acting through a GABA receptor
23. _____ clonazepam (Klonopin)	b. drugs delaying an influx of sodium across neuronal membranes
24. _____ phenytoin (Dilantin)	c. drugs delaying an influx of calcium across neuronal membranes
25. _____ gabapentin (Neurontin)	
26. _____ carbamazepine (Tegretol)	d. amino acid drug compounds
27. _____ ethosuximide (Zarontin)	

MULTIPLE CHOICE

28. What common concern occurs with phenobarbital (Luminal)?

    a. Irregular heartbeat

    b. Blood cell reactions

    c. Hypotension

    d. Vitamin D and folate deficiency

29. What is the main advantage of using carbamazepine (Tegretol) for partial seizures?

    a. Category C status

    b. Dual use for the treatment of trigeminal neuralgia

    c. Ability to cause less drowsiness

    d. Dual use for the treatment of manic-depressive disorder

30. Which one of the following is the more recent hydantoin-like drug?

    a. Phenytoin (Dilantin)

    b. Zonisamide (Zonegran)

    c. Carbamazepine (Tegretol)

    d. Valproic acid (Depakene)

31. Which of the following medications is used to treat Lennox–Gastaut syndrome?

    a. Fosphenytoin (Cerebyx)

    b. Felbamate (Felbatol)

    c. Lamotrigine (Lamictal)

    d. Methsuximide (Celontin)

32. Which antiseizure medication might produce psychotic behavior symptoms?

    a. Ethosuximide (Zarontin)

    b. Mephobarbital (Mebaral)

    c. Lorazepam (Ativan)

    d. Gabapentin (Neurontin)

33. Which is the most potent benzodiazepine used for the treatment of convulsions?

    a. Clonazepam (Klonopin)

    b. Clorazepate (Tranxene)

    c. Diazepam (Valium)

    d. Lorazepam (Ativan)

34. Which of the following medications is converted to phenytoin in the body?

    a. Fosphenytoin (Cerebyx)

    b. Felbamate (Felbatol)

    c. Divalproex (Depakote)

    d. Lamotrigine (Lamictal)

35. What is the major concern in making antiseizure therapy successful?

    a. Avoiding kidney and liver toxicity

    b. Making sure the patient complies with medication

    c. Maintaining proper drug levels in the bloodstream

    d. All of the above

36. Why should women of childbearing age be counseled regarding antiseizure medications?

    a. They are teratogenic.

    b. They interfere with oral contraceptives.

    c. They produce folic acid deficiency.

    d. All of the above

37. Patients taking barbiturates for seizures must be monitored for respiratory depression in the presence of which of the following?

    a. Oral administration

    b. Nonopiate analgesics

    c. Chronic respiratory dysfunction

    d. All of the above

38. A patient is admitted with an overdose of Valium. Which of the following drugs would the nurse need to have on hand?

    a. Diphenhydramine (Benadryl)

    b. Flumazenil (Romazicon)

    c. Epinephrine

    d. Atropine

39. The nurse should teach the patient taking benzodiazepines that the drug can do which of the following?

    a. Cause sedation when first started

    b. Be safely stopped abruptly

    c. Increase the amount of digoxin needed

    d. Be potentiated by smoking, nicotine patches, or chewing tobacco

40. A patient taking phenytoin (Dilantin) chronically for seizures should be encouraged to maintain good oral hygiene and visit the dentist every 6 months. Phenytoin does which of the following in patients?

    a. Causes cavities

    b. Causes gingival hyperplasia

    c. Causes mouth cancers

    d. Builds up tartar on the teeth

MAKING CONNECTIONS

41. Although phenobarbital is an antiseizure medicine, it is also classified as which of the following?

    a. Benzodiazepine

    b. Category I drug

    c. Sympathomimetic

    d. Sedative-hypnotic

42. Which term describes a craving of a patient to continue drug use despite its negative effects?

    a. Tolerance

    b. Physical dependence

    c. Psychological dependence

    d. Resistance

43. When are seizures in a patient who is undergoing alcohol withdrawal most likely to occur?

    a. Immediately after the patient has stopped drinking

    b. 1 to 3 days after the patient has stopped drinking

    c. 5 to 7 days after the patient has stopped drinking

    d. During an episode of delirium tremens (DTs)

44. Which of the following drugs is NOT used to treat convulsions?

    a. Buspirone (BuSpar)

    b. Phenobarbital (Luminal)

    c. Gabapentin (Neurontin)

    d. Carbamazepine (Tegretol)

45. What is the most important reason that benzodiazepines are not used for chronic seizure control?

    a. Tendency for the patient to develop tolerance to the drug

    b. Psychological addiction

    c. Respiratory depression that occurs in chronic use

    d. No antidote exists

CALCULATIONS

46. The physician orders phenobarbital elixir 60 mg PO bid. The pharmacy fills the prescription with phenobarbital elixir 20 mg/5 mL. The patient's care provider should be instructed to administer _____ mL per dose.

47. The physician orders felbamate (Felbatol) 1,200 mg per day in four divided doses. The nurse would give _____ mg per dose.

CASE STUDY APPLICATIONS

48. A nurse is preparing for a patient who is coming to the emergency department with status epilepticus. The physician has ordered phenytoin (Dilantin) by IV drip as soon as the patient arrives.

    a. What evidence (assessment data) would support a nursing diagnosis of *Risk for Injury*?

    b. What interventions would provide safety for the patient during Dilantin administration?

49. A male patient has been placed on phenytoin (Dilantin) for newly diagnosed epilepsy. He has generalized tonic-clonic seizures. He has asked how long it will take to manage his seizures and what side effects can occur. He also wants to know what foods or drugs to avoid while on this medication.

    a. Which nursing diagnosis would be top priority for this patient?

    b. What interventions would be helpful for this diagnosis?

CHAPTER 16

DRUGS FOR EMOTIONAL, MOOD, AND BEHAVIORAL DISORDERS

FILL IN THE BLANK

From the textbook, find the correct word(s) to complete the statement(s).

1. A type of mood disorder experienced by some patients during dark winter months is _____ _____ _____.

2. The two major types of mood disorders are _____ _____ _____ and _____ _____.

3. The three major classes of antidepressants are _____, _____, and _____.

4. _____ are drugs of choice for clinical depression.

5. Other than the SSRIs, _____ produce fewer cardiovascular side effects and therefore are less dangerous than the MAOIs.

6. Patients taking _____ for bipolar disorder should not be placed on a low-sodium diet.

7. The inability to focus or pay attention is one of the main symptoms of _____ _____ _____.

8. _____ is the class of drugs most widely prescribed for ADHD.

9. Drugs for bipolar disorders are called _____ _____ because they have the ability to modulate extreme shifts in emotions between _____ and _____.

Adams/Holland, *Student Workbook and Resource Guide for Pharmacology for Nurses* 4th Edition
© 2014 by Pearson Education, Inc.

MATCHING

For questions 10 through 21, match the drug in column I with its primary indication or class in column II.

Column I	Column II
10. _____ lithium (Eskalith)	a. ADD/CNS stimulant
11. _____ venlafaxine (Effexor)	b. depression/tricyclic type
12. _____ paroxetine (Paxil, Pexeva)	c. depression/MAOI
13. _____ amitriptyline (Elavil)	d. depression/SSRI
14. _____ phenelzine (Nardil)	e. depression/atypical/SNRI
15. _____ methylphenidate (Ritalin)	f. bipolar disorder
16. _____ lisdexamfetamine (Vyvanse)	
17. _____ tranylcypromine (Parnate)	
18. _____ nortriptyline (Aventyl, Pamelor)	
19. _____ bupropion (Wellbutrin, Zyban)	
20. _____ fluoxetine (Prozac)	
21. _____ sertraline (Zoloft)	

For questions 22 through 26, match the definition in column I with its correct term in column II.

Column I	Column II
22. _____ enzyme that breaks down catecholamine neurotransmitters in the synapse	a. amphetamines
23. _____ accumulation of serotonin when taking two drugs that reduce serotonin uptake	b. bipolar disorder
24. _____ condition exhibiting signs of both clinical depression and mania	c. monoamine oxidase
25. _____ the class of drug that is closely related to methylphenidate	d. tyramine
26. _____ chemical found in medications that cannot be ingested by patients on MAOIs because of high risk of severe hypertension	e. serotonin syndrome

MULTIPLE CHOICE

27. What is the most common age range for the diagnosis of attention-deficit disorder (ADD)?

    a. 0 to 3 years

    b. 3 to 7 years

    c. 10 to 13 years

    d. 15 to 18 years

28. Which medication has NOT been useful in stabilizing emotions in mood disorders such as bipolar disorder?

    a. Lithium (Eskalith)

    b. Carbamazepine (Tegretol)

    c. Valproic acid (Depakene, Depakote)

    d. Pemoline (Cylert)

29. Lithium is used with other medications during phases of bipolar disorder. The nurse knows that which of these medications would NOT be used with lithium?

    a. Tricyclic antidepressants

    b. Benzodiazepines

    c. SSRI antidepressants

    d. Diuretics

30. Which of the following is an advantage of using atomoxetine (Strattera) instead of a scheduled CNS stimulant?

    a. Strattera improves ability to focus and decreases hyperactivity.

    b. Strattera has shown more efficacy than Ritalin.

    c. Strattera has fewer CNS side effects than Ritalin.

    d. Strattera is not as addictive as Ritalin.

31. A patient is sent home after being given fluoxetine (Prozac) for depression. The nurse should instruct the patient to do which of the following?

    a. Call back if there is no improvement in 24 hours.

    b. Call back if any nausea, drowsiness, or dizziness occurs.

    c. Start the Prozac before stopping the patient's present MAOI.

    d. Expect to see improvement in mood, appetite, and energy within 1 to 3 weeks.

32. Methylphenidate (Ritalin) produces its effects by activating what portion of the brain?

    a. Cerebellum

    b. Hypothalamus

    c. Pituitary

    d. Reticular activating system

33. When sending a patient home on imipramine (Tofranil), which of the following is important for the nurse to teach patients?

   a. St. John's wort may be used concurrently with no anticipated interaction.

   b. Photosensitivity is not a problem with Tofranil.

   c. This drug should not be stopped abruptly.

   d. Use of this drug with other CNS depressants is permitted.

34. Which of the following is NOT a common symptom of clinical depression?

   a. Lack of energy

   b. Sleep disturbances

   c. Hallucinations

   d. Feelings of despair or guilt

35. In assessing a patient, the nurse should know that rapid shifts in emotions from profound depression to euphoria and hyperactivity are characteristic of which of the following?

   a. Psychosis

   b. Bipolar disorder

   c. Schizophrenia

   d. ADD

36. Which of the following would least likely be used to treat clinical depression?

   a. Monoamine oxidase inhibitors

   b. Tricyclic antidepressants

   c. Selective serotonin reuptake inhibitors

   d. Phenothiazines

37. How does phenelzine (Nardil) produce its therapeutic effects?

   a. Inhibits the reuptake of norepinephrine into presynaptic nerve terminals

   b. Irreversibly inhibits monoamine oxidase (MAO) and intensifies the effects of norepinephrine in the synapse

   c. Selectively inhibits the reuptake of serotonin into presynaptic nerve terminals

   d. Interferes with the binding of dopamine to receptors located in the limbic system

38. How do tricyclic antidepressants produce their therapeutic effects?

   a. Inhibit the reuptake of both serotonin and norepinephrine into presynaptic nerve terminals

   b. Irreversibly inhibit monoamine oxidase (MAO) and intensify the effects of norepinephrine in the synapse

   c. Selectively inhibit the reuptake of serotonin into presynaptic nerve terminals

   d. Interfere with the binding of dopamine to receptors located in the limbic system

39. How does fluoxetine (Prozac) produce its therapeutic effects?

    a. Inhibits the reuptake of both serotonin and norepinephrine into presynaptic nerve terminals

    b. Irreversibly inhibits monoamine oxidase (MAO) and intensifies the effects of norepinephrine in the synapse

    c. Selectively inhibits the reuptake of serotonin into presynaptic nerve terminals

    d. Interferes with the binding of dopamine to receptors located in the limbic system

40. Why are the selective serotonin reuptake inhibitors (SSRIs) generally preferred over other classes of antidepressants?

    a. More efficacious

    b. Produce fewer sympathomimetic and anticholinergic side effects

    c. Do not produce sexual dysfunction

    d. Cause more extrapyramidal effects

41. Because fluoxetine is a chemical precursor for serotonin synthesis, the nurse should teach patients taking fluoxetine to avoid foods high in which amino acid?

    a. Histidine

    b. Tyramine

    c. Lysine

    d. Tryptophan

MAKING CONNECTIONS

42. Typical oral doses are 1 mg for risperidone and 50 mg for clozapine. Which of the following may the nurse correctly conclude from this information?

    a. Risperidone is more efficacious.

    b. Clozapine is more efficacious.

    c. Risperidone is more potent.

    d. Clozapine is more potent.

43. Chlorpromazine is available by both IM and oral routes. Which would be expected to have a faster onset of action?

    a. IM

    b. Oral

44. In assessing a new patient, the nurse should know that panic attacks, phobias, and obsessive–compulsive disorders are usually treated with which of the following?

    a. Antipsychotic drugs

    b. Antianxiety drugs

    c. Drugs for bipolar disorder

    d. Antidepressants

45. "Speedball" is the street name for a drug combination containing methylphenidate (Ritalin) and which of the following?

    a. Heroin

    b. Marijuana

    c. LSD

    d. Cocaine

46. Methylphenidate is a Schedule II drug. What does this mean?

    a. It may adversely affect the fetus.

    b. It has no therapeutic use.

    c. It has a low abuse potential.

    d. It has a high potential for physical and psychological dependence.

CALCULATIONS

47. The physician orders lithium carbonate 1.2 g PO daily in four divided doses. The pharmacy supplies 300 mg lithium carbonate capsules. The nurse should instruct the patient to take _____ capsule(s) per dose.

48. The physician orders fluoxetine 45 mg PO daily. The pharmacy fills the prescription with fluoxetine oral solution of 20 mg/5 mL. The patient should be instructed to take _____ mL per day.

CASE STUDY APPLICATIONS

49. A patient who has bipolar disorder has been started on lithium. He is also on paroxetine (Paxil), digoxin (Lanoxin), furosemide (Lasix), and potassium supplements for depression, hypertension, and CHF. He has also been on a low-sodium diet.

    a. During the first 3 weeks on lithium, what would the nurse identify as the priority nursing diagnosis?

    b. What assessments would the nurse make in identifying this diagnosis?

    c. What is the patient goal for the first 3 weeks of therapy?

50. A female patient has been started on sertraline (Zoloft) for depression. Upon being admitted, she has been assessed as having episodes of crying, feelings of guilt, insomnia, and suicidal ideation. The nurse needs to monitor the patient for effectiveness, side effects, and potential problems.

    a. Discuss what goals might be assigned the patient and how those goals could be evaluated.

CHAPTER 17

DRUGS FOR PSYCHOSES

FILL IN THE BLANK

From the textbook, find the correct word(s) to complete the statement(s).

1. The most common type of psychosis is _____.

2. Acute psychoses develops in _____ _____ _____, whereas chronic psychoses develops over _____ _____ _____.

3. Atypical antipsychotic drugs are effective for both _____ and _____ symptoms of psychosis.

4. The cause of schizophrenia has not been determined, although several theories have been proposed. There appears to be a _____ _____ to schizophrenia. Another theory suggests that the disorder is caused by _____ _____ _____ in specific brain areas.

5. Positive symptoms include _____, _____, _____, and _____.

6. Negative symptoms include a lack of _____, _____, _____, and _____.

7. Proper diagnosis of positive and negative symptoms is important for selection of the appropriate _____ drugs.

8. Symptoms of schizophrenia are thought to be associated with the _____ receptors in the basal nuclei.

9. Medications that block 65% of D_2 receptors will reduce symptoms of _____. Blocking more than 80% of D_2 receptors will likely cause _____ symptoms.

Adams/Holland, *Student Workbook and Resource Guide for Pharmacology for Nurses* 4th Edition
© 2014 by Pearson Education, Inc.

MATCHING

For questions 10 through 19, match the drug in column I with its primary indication or class in column II.

Column I

10. _____ haloperidol (Haldol)

11. _____ thioridazine (Mellaril)

12. _____ chlorpromazine

13. _____ prochlorperazine

14. _____ olanzapine (Zyprexa)

15. _____ loxapine (Loxitane)

16. _____ clozapine (Clozaril)

17. _____ aripiprazole (Abilify)

18. _____ thiothixene (Navane)

19. _____ risperidone (Risperdal)

Column II

a. psychosis/phenothiazine

b. psychosis/nonphenothiazine

c. psychosis/atypical

d. dopamine system stabilizers

For questions 20 through 28, match the characteristics in column I with their terms and conditions in column II.

Column I

20. _____ a condition in which the patient exhibits symptoms of both schizophrenia and mood disorders

21. _____ firm ideas and beliefs not founded in reality

22. _____ symptoms that are added to normal behavior

23. _____ a term meaning "antipsychotic medications"

24. _____ an extreme suspicion that one is being followed, or that others are trying to harm oneself

25. _____ symptoms that subtract from a normal behavior

26. _____ seeing, hearing, or feeling something that is not there

27. _____ a class of drug that might be used to decrease extrapyramidal effects

28. _____ a movement disorder brought on by medication effects

Column II

a. paranoia

b. delusions

c. hallucinations

d. positive symptoms

e. negative symptoms

f. schizoaffective disorders

g. neuroleptics

h. anticholinergics

i. extrapyramidal effects

MULTIPLE CHOICE

29. Which class of drugs tends to produce severe side effects such as muscle twitching, compulsive motor activity, and a Parkinson-like syndrome?

    a. Barbiturates

    b. Phenothiazines

    c. Benzodiazepines

    d. Serotonin reuptake inhibitors

30. Delusions, hallucinations, disordered communication, and difficulty relating to others are symptoms closely associated with which of the following?

    a. Clinical depression

    b. Bipolar disorder

    c. Schizophrenia

    d. ADD

31. Which term/phrase best describes extrapyramidal side effects?

    a. Paranoid delusions

    b. Profound depression

    c. Seizures

    d. Distorted body movements and muscle spasms

32. Like many antipsychotics, chlorpromazine usually takes how long before its therapeutic effect is achieved?

    a. 2 to 3 days

    b. 2 to 3 weeks

    c. 7 to 8 weeks

    d. More than 6 months

33. Many of the major effects of chlorpromazine can be attributed to which of the following?

    a. Inhibiting the reuptake of both serotonin and norepinephrine into presynaptic nerve terminals

    b. Irreversibly inhibiting monoamine oxidase (MAO) and intensifying the effects of norepinephrine in the synapse

    c. Selectively inhibiting the reuptake of serotonin into presynaptic nerve terminals

    d. Interfering with the binding of dopamine to receptors located throughout the brain

34. Why are atypical antipsychotics sometimes preferred over phenothiazines?

    a. They produce no major adverse effects.

    b. They can treat both positive and negative symptoms of psychosis.

    c. They are much more efficacious.

    d. They can improve symptoms within a few days of initial administration.

35. Nonphenothiazine agents differ from phenothiazine agents in what way?

    a. Nonphenothiazines do not produce as many anticholinergic side effects as phenothiazines.

    b. Nonphenothiazines cause less sedation and fewer anticholinergic side effects than phenothiazines.

    c. Phenothiazines do not produce as many side effects as nonphenothiazines.

    d. Phenothiazines cause less sedation and anticholinergic side effects than nonphenothiazines.

36. Patients on clozapine (Clozaril) must watch carefully for signs of agranulocytosis, which include which of the following?

    a. Dizziness and drowsiness

    b. Appetite increase

    c. Fever and sore throat

    d. Bruises and bleeding

37. A patient who is on a phenothiazine complains of having elevated temperature, sweating, and "not feeling well." For what possible indication should the nurse assess the patient?

    a. Agranulocytosis

    b. Neuroleptic malignant syndrome

    c. Infection that may decrease potency of the medication

    d. Dystonic reaction

38. For a patient who has problems with daily compliance, a drug is available that lasts for 3 weeks. Which drug would be a good choice for this patient?

    a. Haloperidol (Haldol LA)

    b. Olanzapine (Zyprexa)

    c. Chlorpromazine (Thorazine)

    d. Clozapine (Clozaril)

MAKING CONNECTIONS

39. A patient has been prescribed an antipsychotic drug that has a high degree of anticholinergic side effects. Anticholinergic effects include which of the following?

    a. Nervousness and tremors

    b. Restlessness and constant movement of legs

    c. Drying of mouth, sedation, and urinary retention

    d. Headaches, skin rashes, and hallucinations

40. The atypical antipsychotics bind to serotonergic and cholinergic sites throughout the brain. The nurse understands that this would affect which neurotransmitters?

    a. Acetylcholine and serotonin

    b. Serotonin and dopamine

    c. Serotonin and norepinephrine

    d. Acetylcholine and norepinephrine

41. Benzodiazepines are often given with antipsychotic drugs. Which benzodiazepine side effects would create a problem when given with antipsychotic medications?

    a. Drowsiness and dry mouth

    b. Lowered seizure threshold

    c. Hypotension and respiratory depression

    d. Bone marrow depression

42. Patients on herbal supplements must be warned about interactions with other prescribed medications. What herbal preparations are sometimes taken to treat mental illness?

    a. Tryptophan

    b. St. John's wort

    c. Kava

    d. All of the above

43. Schizoaffective disorder is treated with antipsychotic medications and may require antidepressants. Which of the following medications is an antidepressant?

    a. Diazepam (Valium)

    b. Phenytoin (Dilantin)

    c. Chlorpromazine (Thorazine)

    d. Paroxetine (Paxil)

CALCULATIONS

44. The physician orders fluphenazine 15 mg SC. The pharmacy supplies fluphenazine 25 mg/mL. The nurse would administer _____ ml SC.

45. A patient has an order for Seroquel 200 mg/day in divided dosages bid. Seroquel comes in 50 mg tablets. How many tablets would the nurse give per dose? _____

CASE STUDY APPLICATIONS

46. A female patient has been taking chlorpromazine (Thorazine) for about a year. She has been having problems with orthostatic hypotension and akathisia, and has needed to take benztropine mesylate (Cogentin) to avoid dystonic reactions. The physician has decided to change her to clozapine (Clozaril). The patient asks the nurse about the advantages and disadvantages of the new drug. The nurse has chosen *Deficient Knowledge* as the nursing diagnosis for this patient.

    a. What interventions would be used for this diagnosis?

    b. How would the nurse evaluate the outcome of the interventions?

47. A female patient has recently been diagnosed with schizophrenia. She has been placed on haloperidol (Haldol) while hospitalized and has had hallucinations and delusions.

    a. What assessments would the nurse need to complete during the first 3 weeks that the patient is on this medication?

CHAPTER 18

DRUGS FOR THE CONTROL OF PAIN

FILL IN THE BLANK

From the textbook, find the correct word(s) to complete the statement(s).

1. The two general classes of pain medications are the _____ and _____.

2. All nonsteroidal anti-inflammatory drugs (NSAIDs) have _____ and _____ activity, as well as analgesic properties.

3. The type of headache characterized by a tightening of the muscles of the head and neck area due to stress is called a _____ headache.

4. A sensory cue that precedes a migraine is called a/an _____.

5. NSAIDs act by inhibiting pain mediators at the _____ level.

6. The sensation of pain may be increased by _____, _____, and _____.

7. Successful choice of pain therapy is dependent on the _____ and _____ of the pain.

8. The goals of pharmacotherapy for migraine are to _____ the migraine in progress and to _____ migraines from occurring.

9. Two major drug classes used for migraine headaches include _____ and _____ _____. Both of these are _____ agonists.

10. Triptans are 5-HT–selective and are thought to act by constricting _____ _____. They may be administered _____, _____, or _____.

Adams/Holland, *Student Workbook and Resource Guide for Pharmacology for Nurses* 4th Edition
© 2014 by Pearson Education, Inc.

MATCHING

For questions 11 through 22, match the drug in column I with its primary indication/class in column II.

Column I

11. _____ naloxone (Narcan)

12. _____ meperidine (Demerol)

13. _____ meloxicam (Mobic)

14. _____ oxycodone (OxyContin, Oxecta)

15. _____ zolmitriptan (Zomig)

16. _____ nalmefene (Revex)

17. _____ ibuprofen (Advil, Motrin)

18. _____ ergotamine tartrate (Ergostat)

19. _____ oxymorphone (Numorphan)

20. _____ fenoprofen (Nalfon)

21. _____ propranolol (Inderal)

22. _____ amitriptyline (Elavil)

Column II

a. NSAID

b. opioid; moderate efficacy

c. opioid; high efficacy

d. opioid blocker

e. antimigraine agent

For questions 23 through 28, match the description in column I with its related term in column II.

Column I

23. _____ natural or synthetic chemicals providing pain relief

24. _____ dull, throbbing, or aching pain

25. _____ caused by injury to tissues

26. _____ sharp localized pain

27. _____ caused by injury to nerves

28. _____ natural chemicals that relieve pain

Column II

a. nociceptor pain

b. neuropathic pain

c. somatic pain

d. visceral pain

e. opiates

f. opioids

MULTIPLE CHOICE

29. Painful disorders having a strong inflammatory component, such as arthritis, are treated most effectively with which of the following?

    a. NSAIDs

    b. Acetaminophen (Tylenol)

    c. Opioids

    d. Herbal supplements

30. When asked why NSAIDs are better than acetaminophen for arthritis, the health care provider responds, "Compared to aspirin, acetaminophen has _____."

    a. Less analgesic activity

    b. No antipyretic activity

    c. No anti-inflammatory activity

    d. The same effect on blood coagulation

31. Which of the following would be used to treat mild to moderate pain due to inflammation?

    a. Oxycodone (OxyContin)

    b. Meperidine (Demerol)

    c. Ibuprofen (Advil)

    d. Acetaminophen (Tylenol)

32. Why are selective COX-2 inhibitors often prescribed over aspirin?

    a. They are more effective at relieving severe pain.

    b. They are more effective at relieving dull, throbbing pain.

    c. They are less expensive.

    d. They cause fewer side effects.

33. ASA is an abbreviation that refers to which of the following?

    a. Any NSAID

    b. Aspirin

    c. Opioid analgesics

    d. COX-2 inhibitors

34. A health care provider sees an order for aspirin 325 mg once daily. The health care provider knows this medication is given at this dose level for what reason?

    a. To prolong clotting times

    b. To fight infections

    c. To relieve pain

    d. To decrease inflammation

35. When a health care provider is asked to explain why acetaminophen (Tylenol) is used more often than aspirin, the response is that aspirin can cause which of the following?

    a. Dependence

    b. Increased platelet adhesiveness

    c. GI bleeding

    d. CNS depression

36. A mother asks why aspirin should not be given to children and teens. The appropriate reaction by the health care provider is based on the actions of aspirin, which can cause which of the following?

    a. Anticoagulant activity

    b. Reduced incidence of strokes

    c. Reduced risk of colorectal cancer

    d. Increased risk of Reye's syndrome

37. Which of the following drugs is commonly given to heroin addicts during treatment of their drug dependence?

    a. Methadone (Dolophine)

    b. Oxycodone

    c. Morphine

    d. Meperidine (Demerol)

38. Why are opioids often used for pain relief following tooth extractions?

    a. They help the patient sleep.

    b. They do not prolong bleeding time.

    c. They can be taken once a day.

    d. They are more efficacious than other analgesics.

39. A health care provider knows that therapeutic effects of opiates do NOT include which of the following?

    a. Treatment of respiratory depression

    b. Treatment of diarrhea

    c. Relief of severe pain

    d. Suppression of cough reflex

40. A patient comes to the emergency department with an overdose of morphine. What would the priority nursing assessment include?

    a. Dilated pupils

    b. Depressed respiration

    c. Hypertension

    d. Diarrhea

41. For an overdose of opiates, what would the health care provider need to have on hand to counteract the effects?

    a. Dextroamphetamine (Dexedrine)

    b. Phenytoin (Dilantin)

    c. Naloxone (Narcan)

    d. Tramadol (Ultram)

42. A patient comes to the ER with a migraine. The health care provider knows that the patient may have an aura prior to the onset of the headache. What does the aura indicate about the patient?

    a. The patient has taken an overdose of aspirin.

    b. The patient has taken an overdose of opioids.

    c. The patient will soon experience a migraine.

    d. The patient has a high fever.

43. What is the mechanism of action of sumatriptan (Imitrex) and other triptans?

    a. Affect mu receptors

    b. Cause vasoconstriction of cranial arteries

    c. Block prostaglandin synthesis

    d. Block COX-2

MAKING CONNECTIONS

44. Besides an antimigraine agent, what is another use for amitriptyline?

    a. Anticonvulsant

    b. Sedative–hypnotic

    c. Antipsychotic

    d. Antidepressant

45. Ergotamine is a Category X drug, which means what about the drug?

    a. It has a high risk of physical and psychological dependence.

    b. It should never be taken during pregnancy.

    c. It has no therapeutic use.

    d. It is very toxic to the patient.

46. Phenobarbital (Luminal) is a sedative–hypnotic that is also prescribed for which of the following?

    a. Migraines

    b. Marijuana addiction

    c. Seizures

    d. Clinical depression

47. Where would an intrathecal injection of morphine be administered?

    a. Spinal subarachnoid space

    b. Brain

    c. Joint

    d. Abdominal cavity

48. What is the first step in pharmacokinetics?

    a. Metabolism

    b. Absorption

    c. Ingestion

    d. Excretion

CALCULATIONS

49. The physician orders ibuprofen 400 mg PO tid. The pharmacy sends ibuprofen suspension 100 mg/5 mL. The patient should receive _____ mL per dose.

50. The physician orders naloxone HCl 0.4 mg IV bolus. The pharmacy supplies naloxone 0.02 mg/mL. The nurse should administer _____ mL IV bolus.

CASE STUDY APPLICATIONS

51. A male patient presents with severe pain in his joints. The nurse assesses this patient's complaints and recommends a course of treatment. The patient is 75 years old and, other than anxiety and insomnia, appears to be in good health. He is interested in nonpharmacologic control of his pain. He admits to being reluctant to take the oxycodone that the health care provider ordered, because he does not want to "become a crazy addict." The nurse has chosen *Deficient Knowledge* for a nursing diagnosis.

    a. What interventions would be appropriate for this situation?

    b. What outcomes would be evaluated for this patient?

52. A female patient has been experiencing migraine headaches for 2 years. She is now seeking medical assistance because they have become more frequent and painful. She states that it takes six aspirin to relieve the pain once the migraine has started. She has a history of chronic heart failure and hypertension. She has heard that drugs used for migraines are addictive and is interested in a nonpharmacologic solution. The patient is taking the following medications:

    oxycodone terephthalate (Percodan) (as needed)

    verapamil (Calan)

    digoxin (Lanoxin)

    a. The nurse chooses *Altered Comfort: Pain* as the diagnosis. What interventions can be used for this nursing diagnosis?

    b. What patient goals would be included in the care for this patient?

Adams/Holland, *Student Workbook and Resource Guide for Pharmacology for Nurses* 4th Edition
© 2014 by Pearson Education, Inc.

CHAPTER 19

DRUGS FOR LOCAL AND GENERAL ANESTHESIA

FILL IN THE BLANK

From the textbook, find the correct word(s) to complete the statement(s).

1. Because local anesthesia is not always applied to small areas of the body, some local anesthetic treatments are more accurately called _____ anesthesia.

2. The direct injection of a local anesthetic into tissue immediate to a surgical site is called _____ anesthesia.

3. The goal of general anesthesia is to provide a rapid and complete loss of _____.

4. The two major ways to induce general anesthesia are by using _____ agents and _____ agents.

5. Opioids are sometimes given as preoperative medications to counteract _____ _____ _____.

6. Local anesthesia is loss of _____ to a small area without loss of _____.

7. In applying local anesthesia, the method employed depends on _____ and _____ _____ _____ _____.

8. In the area where the local anesthetic is applied, _____ and _____ _____ will temporarily diminish.

9. Drug classes used as adjuncts to anesthesia include _____, _____, _____, _____ _____, _____ _____, _____ and _____.

10. With _____ anesthesia, the dose of inhalation anesthetic can be _____, thus making the procedure safer for the patient.

Adams/Holland, *Student Workbook and Resource Guide for Pharmacology for Nurses* 4th Edition
© 2014 by Pearson Education, Inc.

MATCHING

For questions 11 through 23, match the drug in column I with its classification in column II.

Column I

11. _____ droperidol (Inapsine)

12. _____ benzocaine (Anbesol)

13. _____ bupivacaine (Marcaine)

14. _____ enflurane (Ethrane)

15. _____ diazepam (Valium)

16. _____ lidocaine (Xylocaine)

17. _____ prilocaine (Citanest)

18. _____ fentanyl (Sublimaze, others)

19. _____ promethazine (Phenergan, others)

20. _____ ketamine (Ketalar)

21. _____ isoflurane (Forane)

22. _____ midazolam (Versed)

23. _____ propofol (Diprivan)

Column II

a. ester-type local anesthetic

b. amide-type local anesthetic

c. inhaled anesthetic

d. intravenous anesthetic

e. adjunct to anesthesia

For questions 24 through 32, match the characteristics in column I with their drugs or classes in column II.

Column I

24. _____ prolongs duration of local anesthetic agents

25. _____ most commonly used topical anesthetics

26. _____ may be prescribed for cardiac dysrhythmias

27. _____ type of anesthesia most commonly used in obstetrics during labor and delivery

28. _____ most commonly used injectable local anesthetic

29. _____ most commonly used local anesthetic

30. _____ most abused anesthetic agent

31. _____ major depolarizing neuromuscular blocker

32. _____ most widely used inhalation anesthesia

Column II

a. epinephrine

b. epidural

c. amides

d. benzocaine

e. lidocaine

f. isoflurane (Forane)

g. succinylcholine (Anectine)

h. nitrous oxide

Adams/Holland, *Student Workbook and Resource Guide for Pharmacology for Nurses* 4th Edition
© 2014 by Pearson Education, Inc.

MULTIPLE CHOICE

33. Epinephrine is often added to a local anesthetic. The nurse must monitor for which factors when caring for the patient who is due to receive epinephrine in his anesthetic?

    a. Side effects of increased heart rate and blood pressure

    b. History of cardiac conditions

    c. Vital signs

    d. All of the above

34. Which of the following is NOT a major route for applying local anesthetics?

    a. Epidural

    b. Spinal

    c. Nerve block

    d. Inhalation

35. In administering general anesthetics using balanced anesthesia, the nurse would expect which medication to be administered first?

    a. IV anesthesia

    b. Inhalation anesthesia

    c. Analgesics

    d. Neuromuscular blocking agents

36. Nitrous oxide can be administered safely in patients with which of the following?

    a. Myasthenia gravis

    b. Increased anxiety related to pain or procedures

    c. Increased intracranial pressure

    d. Cardiac disease

37. Why is an alkaline substance such as sodium hydroxide sometimes added to a vial of anesthetic solution?

    a. To provide the environment needed for absorption

    b. To prolong the duration of anesthetic action

    c. To increase the effectiveness of the anesthetic in regions that have extensive local infection or abscesses

    d. To decrease the potential for anaphylaxis

38. Which of the following is a potential early adverse effect from local anesthetics?

    a. Hypertension

    b. Myocardial infarction

    c. Flushing

    d. Restlessness or anxiety

39. Which stage of general anesthesia is called surgical anesthesia because it is the stage in which most surgery occurs?

    a. Stage 1

    b. Stage 2

c. Stage 3

d. Stage 4

40. The PRIMARY reason that nitrous oxide is used in short surgical procedures is that it provides which of the following?

    a. Potent analgesia

    b. Sedation/relaxation

    c. Anti-inflammatory properties

    d. Anti-infective properties

41. Inhaled general anesthetics produce their effect by preventing the flow of which of the following into neurons of the CNS?

    a. Carbohydrates

    b. Lipids

    c. Sodium

    d. Calcium

42. Which of the following is a potential early adverse effect from nitrous oxide?

    a. Restlessness or anxiety

    b. Dysrhythmia

    c. Hypertension

    d. Mania

43. What is the major depolarizing neuromuscular blocker used during surgery?

    a. Succinylcholine (Anectine)

    b. Acetylcholine

    c. Promethazine (Phenergan)

    d. Bethanechol (Urecholine)

44. Which of the following is a parasympathomimetic sometimes administered to stimulate the smooth muscle of the bowel and the urinary tract following surgery?

    a. Succinylcholine (Anectine)

    b. Acetylcholine

    c. Promethazine (Phenergan)

    d. Bethanechol (Urecholine)

45. Halothane hepatitis can be prevented by using halothane:

    a. in those presently not pregnant.

    b. at least 21 days apart.

    c. with caution in those having diminished hepatic function.

    d. with caution in those having high blood pressure or irregular heartbeats.

MAKING CONNECTIONS

46. In addition to its use as an injected anesthetic, what is lorazepam (Ativan) also used to treat?

    a. Depression

    b. Anxiety

    c. Loss of appetite

    d. Bipolar disorder

47. Where are sublingual medications administered?

    a. Into a body cavity

    b. Into the subarachnoid spinal space

    c. Into a vein or artery

    d. Under the tongue

48. Which of the following is a hallucinogen?

    a. Psilocybin

    b. Cocaine

    c. Heroin

    d. Marijuana

49. Before administering an opioid, which of the following should be checked?

    a. Blood pressure

    b. Respiration rate

    c. Body temperature

    d. Pulse rate

50. Adrenergic blockers produce a response similar to that of which of the following?

    a. Sympathetic stimulation

    b. Parasympathetic stimulation

    c. Dopaminergic inhibition

    d. Serotonin inhibition

CALCULATIONS

51. Atropine grains 1/6 subcutaneous is ordered. Availability is 15 mg/mL. How many milliliters would be given?

52. Trimethobenzamide (Tigan) 100 mg is ordered IM stat. Availability is an ampule with 200 mg/2 mL. How many milliliters would be given?

CASE STUDY APPLICATIONS

53. A female patient is to undergo a procedure that requires general anesthesia. She asks the nurse what to expect from the medications before and after the procedure.

    a. Identify the nursing diagnosis.

    b. Describe interventions that would be appropriate for this patient.

54. A female patient is to have a minor procedure on her foot during which local anesthesia is to be used. She is anxious and asks how this procedure is done. She asks what type of effect the anesthesia will have and how long the anesthesia will last. The patient has rapid speech and talks in a pressured speech pattern. She is tremulous and seems to be restless, scanning the room frequently.

    a. Identify the nursing diagnosis.

    b. What assessment data would cause the nurse to have chosen this diagnosis?

    c. Describe interventions that would be appropriate for this patient.

    d. Identify the goal(s) for this patient.

    e. How would each goal be evaluated by the nurse?

CHAPTER 20

DRUGS FOR DEGENERATIVE DISEASES OF THE NERVOUS SYSTEM

FILL IN THE BLANK

From the textbook, find the correct word(s) to complete the statement(s).

1. Drug therapy of Parkinson's disease focuses on restoring _____ function and also blocking the effect of _____ within the same area of the brain.

2. _____ _____ is a degenerative disorder characterized by progressive memory loss, confusion, and inability to think or communicate effectively.

3. The etiology of most neurologic degenerative diseases is _____.

4. Patients with Alzheimer's disease experience a dramatic loss of their ability to perform tasks that require _____ as a neurotransmitter.

5. Parkinson's disease could be related to a _____ link because many patients have a family history of the disorder.

6. Extensive treatment with certain _____ medications may induce Parkinson-like syndrome or _____ symptoms.

7. Side effects of drugs used to treat Parkinsonism include _____ and _____. Signs of toxicity would include _____ _____ and _____ _____.

8. When treating Alzheimer's disease, the goal of pharmacotherapy is to improve the function in three domains: _____, _____, and _____ _____ _____ _____.

9. _____ _____ can only be used in the early stages of Alzheimer's because they are only effective in the presence of _____ neurons.

Adams/Holland, *Student Workbook and Resource Guide for Pharmacology for Nurses* 4th Edition
© 2014 by Pearson Education, Inc.

MATCHING

For questions 10 through 19, match the drug in column I with its primary classification in column II.

Column I

10. _____ biperiden (Akineton)

11. _____ levodopa-carbidopa-entacapone (Stalevo)

12. _____ tacrine (Cognex)

13. _____ ropinirole (Requip)

14. _____ benztropine (Cogentin)

15. _____ donepezil (Aricept)

16. _____ bromocriptine (Parlodel)

17. _____ tolcapone (Tasmar)

18. _____ procyclidine (Kemadrin)

19. _____ galantamine (Razadyne, Reminyl)

Column II

a. dopaminergic drug

b. cholinergic blocking drug

c. cholinergic drug (acetylcholinesterase [AChE] inhibitor)

For questions 20 through 28, match the characteristics in column I with their drugs in column II.

Column I

20. _____ decreases effect of dopaminergics

21. _____ antioxidant possibly useful in Alzheimer's disease

22. _____ approved in Europe for dementia but not yet in the United States; can react with anticoagulants

23. _____ antiviral that releases dopamine from its nerve terminals

24. _____ AChE inhibitor used for Alzheimer's disease that is associated with hepatotoxicity

25. _____ drug of choice for Parkinsonism

26. _____ inhibits enzymes that destroy levodopa or dopamine

27. _____ dopamine agonist that activates the dopamine receptors

28. _____ carbidopa that is added to levodopa to make more levodopa available to enter the CNS

Column II

a. levodopa

b. carbodopa-levodopa (Parcopa, Sinemet)

c. selegiline (Eldepryl, Zelapar)

d. bromocriptine (Parlodel)

e. amantadine (Symmetrel)

f. tacrine (Cognex)

g. Ginkgo biloba

h. donepezil (Aricept)

i. pyridoxine (vitamin B_6)

MULTIPLE CHOICE

29. Parkinson's disease is a degenerative disorder of the nervous system caused by the death of neurons that produce which of the following?

    a. Dopamine

    b. Norepinephrine

    c. Acetylcholine

    d. Serotonin

30. A patient is admitted with a new diagnosis of Parkinson's disease. If he is in the early stages, what would usually NOT be seen on assessment?

    a. Tremor

    b. Muscle rigidity and weakness

    c. Bradykinesia

    d. Dementia

31. What is the relationship between acetylcholine and dopamine in the area of the brain that affects balance, posture, and involuntary muscle movement?

    a. Both dopamine and acetylcholine stimulate this region.

    b. Both dopamine and acetylcholine inhibit this region.

    c. Dopamine stimulates and acetylcholine inhibits this region.

    d. Dopamine inhibits and acetylcholine stimulates this region.

32. What class of drugs may induce artificial parkinsonism by interfering with the same neural pathway and functions modified by a lack of dopamine?

    a. Phenothiazines

    b. Tricyclic antidepressants

    c. MAO inhibitors

    d. Benzodiazepines

33. A patient develops extrapyramidal symptoms (EPS) after taking phenothiazines. The nurse would expect an order for which medication to counteract the EPS?

    a. Diphenhydramine (Benadryl)

    b. Procyclidine (Kemadrin)

    c. Levodopa (Larodopa)

    d. Tacrine (Cognex)

34. Which drug has been prescribed more extensively than any other drug for patients with Parkinson's disease?

    a. Carbidopa (Lodosyn)

    b. Benztropine (Cogentin)

    c. Levodopa (Larodopa)

    d. Tacrine (Cognex)

35. A patient is started on levodopa for Parkinson's disease. What type of side effects would be expected?

    a. Sleep disorders such as insomnia

    b. Sedation

    c. Involuntary muscle movements

    d. Seizures

36. If a patient is unable to tolerate dopaminergic medications, which class of drugs would likely be prescribed?

    a. Cholinergic drugs

    b. Anticholinergic drugs

    c. Antipsychotic drugs

    d. Selective serotonin reuptake inhibitors (SSRIs)

37. What normally causes vascular dementia?

    a. Multiple strokes

    b. Multiple heart attacks

    c. Too little blood flow to the brain

    d. Lack of sufficient neurotransmitters in certain areas of the brain

38. Amyloid plaques and neurofibrillary tangles within the brain are diagnostic signs of which of the following?

    a. Parkinson's disease

    b. Tardive dyskinesia

    c. Vascular dementia

    d. Alzheimer's disease

39. Acetylcholine inhibitors enhance the action of what chemical in the brain?

    a. Dopamine

    b. Norepinephrine

    c. Acetylcholine

    d. Serotonin

40. Drugs that inhibit the enzyme AChE will do which of the following?

    a. Increase levels of dopamine

    b. Decrease levels of dopamine

    c. Increase levels of acetylcholine

    d. Decrease levels of acetylcholine

41. When a patient takes phenothiazines for an extended time, what conditions would the nurse expect to see?

    a. Parkinsonism

    b. Hypertensive crisis

    c. Decreased muscle rigidity

    d. Bruising and bleeding from the gums

MAKING CONNECTIONS

42. An anticholinergic drug is one that blocks the effects of which of the following?

    a. Epinephrine

    b. Norepinephrine

    c. Acetylcholine

    d. Serotonin

43. Succinimides, barbiturates, and benzodiazepines are used to treat what disorder?

    a. Anxiety

    b. Seizures

    c. Sleep disorders

    d. Mood disorders

44. Tacrine (Cognex) is highly metabolized by the liver. During the process of metabolism, what happens to the medication?

    a. It is absorbed into the bloodstream.

    b. It is excreted from the body.

    c. It is added to plasma proteins.

    d. It is made more or less inactive.

45. Which type of drug is given to discourage tardive dyskinesias in patients being treated for psychosis?

    a. Cholinergic

    b. Anticholinergics

    c. Dopaminergics

    d. Selective serotonin uptake inhibitors

46. Antipsychotic medications have actions that decrease which of the following in the brain?

    a. Dopamine

    b. Acetylcholine

    c. Norepinephrine

    d. AChE

CALCULATIONS

47. A patient has an order for tolcapone (Tasmar) 100 mg tid. The drug is available in 25-mg tablets. How many tablets would the nurse give per day?

48. A patient has an order for trihexyphenidyl (Artane) 7.5 mg per day. He is to take it tid. He should take _____ mg/dose.

CASE STUDY APPLICATIONS

49. A 30-year-old male patient has recently been diagnosed with early Parkinson's disease. He has been quite upset and depressed about the diagnosis and has lost interest in most of his usual activities and hobbies. His wife reports that his tremors and involuntary movements have worsened. He has been taking the following medications for 6 months: levodopa (2 g/day) and sertraline (Zoloft). He now has benztropine mesylate (Cogentin) added to his medications.

    a. What is the nursing diagnosis that best describes problems related to his condition and his new medication?

    b. What goal would relate to the diagnosis?

50. A male patient has been brought to your facility by the patient's wife. He was diagnosed last year with Alzheimer's disease. His confusion has become increasingly worse. He has been restless, agitated, and experiencing hallucinations. This past year, he has been taking moderate doses of amitriptyline (Elavil) and alprazolam (Xanax). The patient is now placed on donepezil (Aricept) for a trial. During the first 4 weeks of the treatment with this AChE inhibitor, monitoring for adverse reactions and effectiveness is the nurse's responsibility.

    a. What would be the priority nursing diagnosis for this situation?

    b. What interventions would be included?

CHAPTER 21

DRUGS FOR NEUROMUSCULAR DISORDERS

FILL IN THE BLANK

From the textbook, find the correct word(s) to complete the statement(s).

1. Disorders associated with _____ are some of the most difficult conditions to treat because of their underlying mechanisms.

2. Movement disorders span the _____, _____, _____, and _____ body systems.

3. Involuntary contractions of a muscle or group of muscles are called _____ _____.

4. Pharmacotherapy used for muscle spasm usually includes _____, _____ _____, and _____ drugs.

5. A muscle condition that results from damage to the CNS is _____.

6. A chronic neurologic disorder in which involuntary muscle contraction forces body parts into abnormal postures is _____.

7. A single prolonged muscle spasm is referred to as _____ _____.

Adams/Holland, *Student Workbook and Resource Guide for Pharmacology for Nurses* 4th Edition
© 2014 by Pearson Education, Inc.

MATCHING

For questions 8 through 15, match the drug in column I with the letter for the drug classification in column II.

Column I

8. _____ cyclobenzaprine (Amrix, Flexeril)

9. _____ dantrolene (Dantrium)

10. _____ onabotulinumtoxinA (Botox, Dysport)

11. _____ diazepam (Valium)

12. _____ chlorzoxazone (Paraflex, Parafon Forte)

13. _____ rimabotulinumtoxinB (Myobloc)

14. _____ carisoprodol (Soma)

15. _____ methocarbamol (Robaxin)

Column II

a. centrally acting antispasmodic

b. skeletal muscle relaxer (direct-acting antispasmodic)

MULTIPLE CHOICE

16. Causes of muscle spasms include all EXCEPT:

    a. overmedication with antipsychotic drugs.

    b. overdose of calcium.

    c. hypocalcemia.

    d. epilepsy.

17. Nonpharmacologic measures that may be used to treat muscle spasms include all EXCEPT:

    a. encouraging use of the affected muscle.

    b. thermotherapy.

    c. hydrotherapy.

    d. ultrasound.

18. Which of the following statements about cyclobenzaprine (Amrix, Flexeril) is false?

    a. Its mechanism of action is similar to that of tricyclic antidepressants.

    b. It is effective in cerebral palsy.

    c. It is meant for short-term use.

    d. It is not recommended for use in children.

19. All of the following drugs are effective in the treatment of spasticity EXCEPT:

    a. baclofen (Lioresal).

    b. diazepam (Valium).

    c. dantrolene (Dantrium).

    d. cyclobenzaprine (Amrix, Flexeril).

20. How does onabotulinumtoxinA (Botox, Dysport) produce its effects?

    a. It blocks the release of norepinephrine from nerve tissue.

    b. It blocks the release of acetylcholine from cholinergic nerve terminals.

    c. It increases the release of acetylcholine from cholinergic nerve terminals.

    d. It increases the rate at which GABA is broken down in the body.

21. When teaching a patient receiving a centrally acting antispasmodic drug, which statement is NOT correct?

    a. "You should avoid hazardous activities such as driving if the drug makes you drowsy."

    b. "You should avoid alcohol and antihistamines."

    c. "If you have severe side effects, stop taking the drug at once."

    d. "You should not take this drug if you have liver disease."

22. All of the following statements regarding dantrolene (Dantrium) are correct EXCEPT:

    a. its use is contraindicated in patients with malignant hyperthermia.

    b. it is useful in spasms of head and neck muscles.

    c. it is useful in cases of spinal cord injury or CVA.

    d. it does not affect cardiac or smooth muscle.

23. Neuromuscular blockers of the depolarizing blocking type are used primarily for:

    a. patients receiving electroconvulsive therapy (ECT).

    b. shorter surgical procedures.

    c. longer surgical procedures.

    d. both a and b.

24. Which of these drugs is produced by bacteria and is responsible for food poisoning in high quantities?

    a. Dantrolene (Dantrium)

    b. OnabotulinumtoxinA (Botox, Dysport)

    c. Clonazepam (Klonopin)

    d. Diazepam (Valium)

25. Which of the following drug classes increases the risk of unfavorable reactions to antispasmodics?

    a. MAO inhibitors

    b. Pain medications

    c. Antibiotics

    d. Anticonvulsants

26. Baclofen (Lioresal) may be preferred for which of the following reasons?

    a. Less drowsiness and dizziness compared to other antispasmodics

    b. Direct site of action at the neuromuscular junction

    c. Wide safety margin

    d. Both a and b

27. A patient reports to the nurse that, in addition to the drug therapy provided by his health care provider, he is using cayenne (*Capsicum annum*) for his muscle spasms. Which precaution should this patient take?

    a. Wear sun block lotion and long sleeves.

    b. Never apply to broken skin.

    c. Do not use this substance if you use any alcohol.

    d. If you notice any urinary hesitancy, discontinue use at once.

MAKING CONNECTIONS

28. What is the neurotransmitter for skeletal muscle contraction?

    a. Acetylcholine

    b. Serotonin

    c. Norepinephrine

    d. Epinephrine

29. Which physiological action other than sympathomimetic activation depends on norepinephrine?

    a. Appropriate learning and memory

    b. Normal firing of neurons

    c. Proper muscle movements

    d. Stable mood and emotional functioning

30. Dopamine is synthesized naturally from which of the following precursors?

    a. Choline

    b. Tyrosine

    c. Trytophan

    d. Pyruvate

31. Which of the following neurotransmitters is also known as 5-hydroxytryptamine?

    a. Dopamine

    b. Serotonin

    c. *N*-Methyl-D-aspartate

    d. Norepinephrine

32. Which of the following statements about NSAIDs is false?

    a. They are used to decrease inflammation after injuries.

    b. They include aspirin, ibuprofen, naproxen, and acetaminophen.

    c. One of their main side effects is GI upset.

    d. They are used to treat fever.

CALCULATIONS

33. The patient has an order for dantrolene (Dantrium) 75 mg bid. On hand are tablets labeled "dantrolene 25 mg." How many tablets should the nurse give for each dose? How many milligrams will the nurse give per day?

34. The patient has an order for cyclobenzaprine (Flexeril) 20 mg tid. On hand are tablets labeled "cyclobenzaprine 10 mg." How many tablets should the nurse give for each dose? Is this a safe dose?

CASE STUDY APPLICATIONS

35. A female patient has been experiencing lower back pain for 2 months due to muscle spasms. So far, no other disorders have been identified that could explain this pain. Her health care provider has prescribed cyclobenzaprine (Flexeril).

    a. Describe other nondrug therapy that might help in this case.

    b. When teaching the patient about adverse reactions to cyclobenzaprine, what information should be included?

    c. How will the nurse determine whether this drug is effective?

    d. Prior to discharge, the nurse's goal is to have the patient state ways to prevent recurrence of her symptoms. What preventive teaching should be done for this patient?

36. A female patient's career is as a model and fashion designer. She expresses concern over the "crow's feet and frown lines" she is beginning to develop. She asks for information on the new Botox injections she has heard about. She expresses concern over the fact that she's heard they use a "poison" to remove facial wrinkles but says, "It would be great to look 16 again!" The nurse chooses the nursing diagnosis of *Deficient Knowledge* related to use of cosmetic procedures, and teaching is a planned intervention.

    a. What misinformation does the nurse need to correct when talking with this patient?

    b. What side effects does the patient need to be aware of before having the Botox injections?

37. A 21-year-old patient with cerebral palsy is cared for at home by his parents. His mother expresses concern over his spasticity and wants "better drugs" to control it. He is currently using baclofen (Lioresal).

    a. What assessments should be done on this patient?

    b. What nondrug therapy might be useful for this patient?

    c. What patient/family teaching should be done regarding this patient's use of antispasmodic drugs at home?

    d. What patient/family teaching should be done regarding nondrug and safety interventions for this patient?

CHAPTER 22

DRUGS FOR LIPID DISORDERS

FILL IN THE BLANK

From the textbook, find the correct word(s) to complete the statement(s).

1. The general term that means high levels of lipids in the blood is _____.

2. Cholesterol contributes to the fatty _____ that narrows arteries.

3. The three basic types of lipids are _____, _____, and _____.

4. Lipoproteins consist of various amounts of _____, _____, and _____ plus a protein carrier.

5. The _____ class of drugs interferes with a critical enzyme in the synthesis of cholesterol.

Adams/Holland, *Student Workbook and Resource Guide for Pharmacology for Nurses* 4th Edition
© 2014 by Pearson Education, Inc.

MATCHING

For questions 6 through 9, match the drug in column I with its primary class in column II.

Column I	Column II
6. _____ cholestyramine (Questran)	a. HMG-CoA reductase inhibitor
7. _____ niacin	b. bile acid sequestrant
8. _____ gemfibrozil (Lopid)	c. fibric acid agent
9. _____ atorvastatin (Lipitor)	d. none of the above

MULTIPLE CHOICE

10. Drugs that lower blood lipid levels are intended to reduce the likelihood of which of the following?

    a. Dysrhythmias

    b. Colon cancer

    c. Coronary artery disease

    d. Obesity

11. LDL transports cholesterol from the liver to the tissues and organs, where it is used to do which of the following?

    a. Provide energy for cells

    b. Build plasma membranes or to synthesize steroids

    c. Make bile

    d. Make HDL

12. Because the LDLs contribute significantly to plaque deposits, it is often called what type of cholesterol?

    a. Good

    b. Bad

    c. High

    d. Low

13. What happens to the cholesterol component of HDL after it is transported to the liver?

    a. It is used to make LDLs.

    b. It is used to build plasma membranes.

    c. It is used as an energy source.

    d. It is broken down to become part of bile.

14. Which of the following is NOT a lifestyle change that should be considered by patients with high blood lipid levels?

    a. Maintain weight at an optimum level

    b. Implement a medically supervised exercise plan

    c. Reduce sources of stress

    d. Limit soluble fiber in the diet to 2 or fewer grams per day

15. Which of the following should the nurse monitor carefully during the first few months of therapy with statins?

    a. Blood pressure

    b. Sleep patterns

    c. Cardiac function

    d. Liver function

16. The nurse understands that bile acid sequestrants produce their therapeutic effects by doing which of the following?

    a. Inhibiting HMG-CoA reductase

    b. Increasing excretion of cholesterol in the feces

    c. Decreasing production of HDL

    d. Decreasing absorption of dietary lipids

17. All of the following are true regarding cholestyramine (Questran) EXCEPT:

    a. it is not absorbed or metabolized once it enters the intestine.

    b. it acts by inhibiting cholesterol biosynthesis.

    c. its most frequent side effects are constipation, bloating, gas, and nausea.

    d. it should not be taken at the same time as other medications.

18. Which of the following is a B-complex vitamin?

    a. Niacin

    b. Gemfibrozil (Lopid)

    c. Lovastatin (Mevacor)

    d. Colestipol (Colestid)

19. Which of the following best describes the use of niacin in treating hyperlipidemias?

    a. It should not be used in patients with hypercholesterolemia.

    b. It should not be used in patients with a history of heart failure.

    c. It should not be used with other antilipidemics, because their effects may cancel each other.

    d. It is most often used in low doses in combination with a statin.

20. Which of the following should be taken separately from other medications, because it may interfere with drug absorption?

    a. Niacin

    b. Gemfibrozil (Lopid)

    c. Cholestyramine (Questran)

    d. Fluvastatin (Lescol)

MAKING CONNECTIONS

21. Which of the following best describes concerns associated with phenelzine (Nardil)?

    a. It should not be taken concurrently with MAOIs.

    b. Patients must avoid foods containing tyramine.

    c. It may affect the therapeutic outcome of some antiseizure mediations.

    d. It may potentiate the effects of anticholinergic drugs.

22. Which of the following is NOT a therapeutic effect of aspirin?

    a. Increases PT time

    b. Prevents heart attack

    c. Relieves severe pain

    d. Reduces inflammation

23. Which of the following medications is used primarily for insomnia therapy?

    a. Zolpidem (Ambien)

    b. Pentobarbital (Nembutal)

    c. Alprazolam (Xanax)

    d. Escitalopram (Lexapro)

24. Which of the following is true regarding category D drugs?

    a. They may be safely used in pregnant patients.

    b. Animal studies indicate some risk, but the drug appears to be safe for humans.

    c. They should only be used in pregnant patients if the potential benefit justifies the potential risk to the fetus.

    d. They should not be used in pregnant patients under any circumstance.

25. Which of the following is used to treat seizures?

    a. Lidocaine (Xylocaine)

    b. Fluoxetine (Prozac)

    c. Valproic acid (Depakote)

    d. Haloperidol (Haldol)

CALCULATIONS

26. The physician orders simvastatin (Zocor) 40 mg at bedtime. The supply is 20-mg tablets scored. How many tablets will the nurse give the patient, and at what time?

27. The nurse practitioner orders gemfibrozil (Lopid) 1.2 g daily in two divided doses. The pharmacy sends several 600-mg scored tablets. How many tablets will the nurse give, and at what time?

CASE STUDY APPLICATIONS

28. A 57-year-old obese male with a history of two heart attacks over the past 3 years has been treated with antihypertensives for hypertension. LDL cholesterol was recently measured at 190 mg/dL and triglycerides were 900 mg/dL. The patient does not smoke and walks 0.25 mile twice a week.

    a. What data can you identify from the initial assessment that would support a nursing diagnosis of *Deficient Knowledge* related to disease process and lifestyle implications of coronary heart disease?

    b. Does the clinical history warrant the implementation of antihyperlipidemic therapy? Why?

    c. Considering this patient's history, what lifestyle suggestions might the nurse offer?

29. A 35-year-old female who is 25 pounds overweight exercises regularly and has been taking 40 mg/day of atorvastatin (Lipitor) for the past 2 years. Although her blood lipid profile was normal 12 months ago, her lipid levels have slowly risen to 1,000 mg/dL (normal 400 to 800 mg/dL).

    a. How does the nurse evaluate this change in lipid level?

    b. What teaching plan would the nurse implement to help these lipid levels return to normal?

CHAPTER 23

DIURETIC THERAPY AND DRUGS FOR RENAL FAILURE

FILL IN THE BLANK

From the textbook, find the correct word(s) to complete the statements(s).

1. Thiazide diuretics act on the _____ tubule of the nephron.

2. Sodium and potassium are exchanged in the _____ tubule, where Na^+ is _____ back into the body and K^+ is _____ into the tubule.

3. Identify the parts of the nephron shown in Figure 23–1.

   A. _____

   B. _____

   C. _____

   D. _____

   E. _____

   F. _____

   G. _____

   H. _____

   I. _____

Adams/Holland, *Student Workbook and Resource Guide for Pharmacology for Nurses* 4th Edition
© 2014 by Pearson Education, Inc.

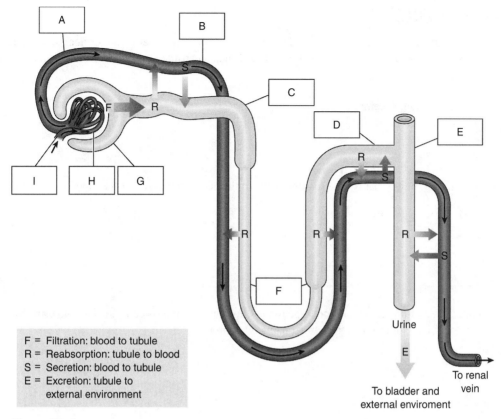

F = Filtration: blood to tubule
R = Reabsorption: tubule to blood
S = Secretion: blood to tubule
E = Excretion: tubule to
      external environment

Figure 23–1.

MATCHING

For questions 4 through 13, match the drug in column I with its classification in column II.

Column I	Column II
4. _____ bumetanide (Bumex)	a. loop diuretic
5. _____ indapamide (Lozol)	b. thiazide or thiazide-like diuretic
6. _____ triamterene (Dyrenium)	c. potassium-sparing diuretic
7. _____ metolazone (Zaroxolyn)	d. carbonic anhydrase inhibitor diuretic
8. _____ mannitol (Osmitrol)	e. osmotic diuretic
9. _____ spironolactone (Aldactone)	
10. _____ acetazolamide (Diamox)	
11. _____ furosemide (Lasix)	
12. _____ eplerenone (Inspra)	
13. _____ hydrochlorothiazide (Microzide)	

MULTIPLE CHOICE

14. The nurse administering diuretics understands that reabsorption and secretion are critical to pharmacokinetics. The composition of the filtrate that passes through Bowman's capsule is similar to which of the following?

    a. Plasma

    b. Plasma minus large proteins

    c. Urine

    d. Blood

15. Medications in the filtrate that pass across the walls of the nephron to re-enter the blood use what process?

    a. Reabsorption

    b. Urination

    c. Secretion

    d. Absorption

16. Drugs, such as penicillin G, that are too large to pass through Bowman's capsule enter the urine by crossing from the peritubular capillaries to the filtrate using what process?

    a. Excretion

    b. Reabsorption

    c. Metabolism

    d. Secretion

17. The nurse explains to the patient that the main function of a diuretic is to increase which of the following?

    a. Reabsorption of water in the nephron

    b. Blood flow through Bowman's capsule

    c. Urine output

    d. Secretion of water in the nephron

18. The nurse understands that most diuretics act by blocking the reabsorption in the nephron of which of the following?

    a. Large proteins

    b. Potassium

    c. Electrolytes

    d. Sodium

19. Which of the following classes of diuretics can cause large amounts of fluid to be excreted by the kidney in a short time when administered IV?

    a. Loop

    b. Thiazides

    c. Osmotic

    d. Potassium sparing

20. Medications that block reabsorption of sodium also affect the amount of water in the filtrate. What effect (if any) does this have on urine flow?

    a. No effect

    b. Increased flow

    c. Decreased flow

    d. Flow may increase or decrease depending on lifestyle factors.

21. The nurse is administering a thiazide diuretic. The nurse should monitor for which common and serious adverse effect of diuretic therapy?

    a. Edema

    b. Hyperkalemia

    c. Dehydration

    d. Hypertension

22. The nurse is administering a loop diuretic. The nurse must monitor for which of the following adverse effects specific to the loop class of diuretics?

    a. Hepatotoxicity

    b. Ototoxicity

    c. Edema

    d. Acidosis

23. Which of the following is the most widely prescribed class of diuretics?

    a. Loop/high-ceiling diuretics

    b. Potassium sparing

    c. Carbonic anhydrase inhibitors

    d. Thiazides

24. The nurse should know that which of the following patients would most likely be administered a thiazide diuretic?

    a. A 50-year-old with mild to moderate hypertension

    b. A 34-year-old with pyelonephritis

    c. An 80-year-old with dehydration

    d. A 60-year-old with lung cancer

25. The nurse teaches the patient that intake of potassium-rich foods should NOT be increased during therapy with which of the following medications?

    a. Furosemide (Lasix)

    b. Chlorothiazide (Diuril)

    c. Spironolactone (Aldactone)

    d. Acetazolamide (Diamox)

26. The nurse is administering 50 mg/day of spironolactone (Aldactone) to a patient with edema. The nurse should know that spironolactone acts by inhibiting which of the following?

    a. Aldosterone

    b. Carbonic anhydrase

    c. Potassium reabsorption in the distal tubule

    d. Sodium reabsorption in the loop of Henle

27. Which diuretic is prescribed specifically to decrease intraocular fluid pressure in patients with open-angle glaucoma?

    a. Torsemide (Demadex)

    b. Triamterene (Dyrenium)

    c. Chlorthalidone (Hygroton)

    d. Acetazolamide (Diamox)

MAKING CONNECTIONS

28. Phenothiazines can cause extrapyramidal symptoms. Which of the following medications may be given to reverse these symptoms?

    a. Benztropine (Cogentin)

    b. Atropine sulfate

    c. Midazolam (Versed)

    d. Naloxone (Narcan)

29. Scopolamine (Transderm-Scop) is an anticholinergic drug primarily used for which of the following?

    a. Dysrhythmias

    b. Hypertension

    c. Inflammation

    d. Motion sickness

30. An overdose of an adrenergic drug is evidenced by which of the following?

    a. Decreased heart rate

    b. Decreased respiratory rate

    c. Increased peristalsis

    d. Dilated pupils

31. Which of the following would NOT be expected from an overdose of an opioid?

    a. CNS depression

    b. Diarrhea

    c. Respiratory depression

    d. Constricted pupils

32. Which of the following drugs is used to dissolve thrombi?

    a. Atenolol (Tenormin)

    b. Warfarin (Coumadin)

    c. Heparin

    d. Reteplase (Retavase)

CALCULATIONS

33. The physician ordered metolazone (Mykrox) 1 mg PO. The pharmacy has 0.5 mg tablets. How many tablets will the nurse administer?

34. The physician ordered acetazolamide (Diamox) 500 mg IVPB added to 100 mL D5W to be infused over 2 hours. The drop factor is 10 gtt/mL. How many gtt/min should be given to infuse the total amount in 2 hours?

CASE STUDY APPLICATIONS

35. An active 56-year-old man was diagnosed with hypertension 12 months ago. At that time, he was placed on verapamil (Calan), hydrochlorothiazide (Microzide), and oral potassium chloride. He has not returned to the office since the initial diagnosis. During the past 12 months, he has reduced his weight from 280 lb to 198 lb using a rigorous exercise and diet program. Although he is proud of his lifestyle changes, he is complaining of fatigue, dizziness, heart palpitations, and muscle weakness.

    a. List two nursing diagnoses appropriate for this patient.

    b. What further assessment data should be obtained?

36. A 49-year-old female television producer works 70 hours per week and has recently been diagnosed with hypertension. The patient reports smoking one pack of cigarettes per day for the past 15 years. She is concerned about the new medication prescribed for her, spironolactone (Aldactone). She appears distressed yet in a hurry to return to work.

    a. What immediate goals are appropriate for this patient?

    b. What patient teaching is appropriate for this patient? Include teaching methods.

CHAPTER 24

DRUGS FOR FLUID BALANCE, ELECTROLYTE, AND ACID–BASE DISORDERS

FILL IN THE BLANK

From the textbook, find the correct word(s) to complete the statements(s).

1. _____ are intravenous (IV) solutions that contain electrolytes that are used to replace lost fluids and to promote urine output.

2. When the body's pH drops below _____, acidosis occurs and symptoms of CNS depression are observed.

3. The normal pH of most body fluids is approximately _____ to _____.

4. Increasing the renal excretion of bicarbonate ion will _____ the pH of the blood.

5. IV fluids that are _____ cause water to move from the interstitial fluid to the plasma.

6. IV fluids that are _____ cause water to move from the plasma to the interstitial fluid.

7. IV fluids that are _____ produce no net fluid shift.

Adams/Holland, *Student Workbook and Resource Guide for Pharmacology for Nurses* 4th Edition
© 2014 by Pearson Education, Inc.

MATCHING

For questions 8 through 12, match the drug in column I with its classification in column II.

Column I	Column II
8. _____ dextran 70 in normal saline	a. colloid
9. _____ 5% dextrose in water (D₅W)	b. crystalloid
10. _____ Plasma-Lyte	
11. _____ hetastarch 6% in normal saline	
12. _____ lactated Ringer's	

MULTIPLE CHOICE

13. The nurse is administering sodium bicarbonate PO 1 g/day. The nurse will begin to recognize symptoms of alkalosis at a pH above which of the following?

    a. 6.5

    b. 7.0

    c. 7.35

    d. 7.45

14. The nurse is assessing for metabolic acidosis. The nurse should first assess for abnormalities in which body system?

    a. GI

    b. CNS

    c. Renal

    d. Cardiovascular

15. The nurse would expect to administer which of the following to a patient with alkalosis?

    a. Sodium bicarbonate

    b. Sodium chloride combined with potassium chloride

    c. Lithium carbonate

    d. Aluminum hydroxide

16. The nurse should know that which of the following is a drug for treating acidosis?

    a. Sodium bicarbonate

    b. Sodium chloride

    c. Ammonium chloride

    d. Potassium chloride

Adams/Holland, *Student Workbook and Resource Guide for Pharmacology for Nurses* 4th Edition
© 2014 by Pearson Education, Inc.

17. When treating hypokalemia, the nurse should know that which of the following is a drug of choice?

    a. Sodium bicarbonate

    b. Sodium chloride

    c. Ammonium chloride

    d. Potassium chloride

18. The nurse should monitor for which of the following common adverse effects of oral potassium chloride when treating a patient for hypokalemia

    a. Drowsiness

    b. Nausea and vomiting

    c. Hypoglycemia

    d. Muscle weakness and fatigue

19. In severe cases, serum potassium levels may be quickly lowered by administration of which of the following?

    a. Glucose and insulin

    b. Furosemide (Lasix)

    c. Acetazolamide (Diamox)

    d. Sodium bicarbonate

20. Colloids cause water molecules to move from the tissues into the blood vessels through their ability to increase which of the following?

    a. Potassium levels

    b. Sodium levels

    c. Sodium excretion

    d. Osmotic pressure

21. Patients who need sodium replacement may be prescribed an IV solution containing which of the following?

    a. Large proteins

    b. Glucose

    c. Electrolytes

    d. Dextran

22. The nurse should know that which of the following patients would most likely suffer from acidosis?

    a. A 70-year-old with kidney failure

    b. A 34-year-old who has ingested excess sodium bicarbonate

    c. A 15-year-old with hyperventilation due to anxiety

    d. A 57-year-old taking diuretics

23. Which of the following situations may lead to alkalosis?

    a. Hypoventilation or shallow breathing

    b. Severe vomiting

    c. Severe diarrhea

    d. Diabetes mellitus

24. The nurse correctly identifies hyponatremia when reviewing which of the following lab values?

    a. Sodium 133 mEq/L

    b. Sodium 148 mEq/L

    c. Potassium 3.5 mEq/L

    d. Potassium 5.5 mEq/L

25. The nurse should teach patients taking potassium supplements to take the drug according to which method?

    a. With no other medications

    b. 1 hour before or 2 hours after a meal

    c. With a meal

    d. In the morning, on awakening

MAKING CONNECTIONS

26. Which of the following antihypertensive drug classes inhibits aldosterone secretion?

    a. ACE inhibitors

    b. Calcium channel blockers

    c. Adrenergic agents

    d. Direct-acting vasodilators

27. An altered physical condition caused by the nervous system adapting to repeated drug use is:

    a. psychological dependence.

    b. physical dependence.

    c. tolerance.

    d. withdrawal.

28. Which of the following is classified as a platelet enhancer?

    a. Folic acid

    b. Epoetin alfa (Epogen, Procrit)

    c. Filgrastim (Neupogen)

    d. Oprelvekin (Neomega)

29. The nurse encourages intake of cranberry juice for a patient with frequent urinary tract infections because cranberries may do which of the following?

    a. Increase the urine acidity

    b. Decrease the urine acidity

    c. Increase hematocrit levels

    d. Decrease hematocrit levels

30. All of the following are used for treating anaphylaxis EXCEPT:

    a. antihistamines.

    b. vasodilators.

    c. corticosteroids.

    d. bronchodilators.

CALCULATIONS

31. The health care provider ordered crystalloid solution 1,000 ml 0.9% NaCl to infuse per pump over 8 hours. The nurse will set the pump at what rate?

32. The physician ordered ammonium chloride 8 g/day in divided doses every 6 h. The pharmacy sends 500-mg tablets. How many tablets will the nurse administer at each dose?

CASE STUDY APPLICATIONS

33. A woman decided to lose weight and chose a plan that eliminated almost all dietary carbohydrates. She has been taking hydrochlorothiazide and aspirin for her arthritis and potassium chloride. After 2 weeks, she can no longer endure the stomach pain, nausea, and cramping. Her husband reports that his wife has shown considerable fatigue and sleepiness.

    a. Analyze the assessment data to develop a nursing plan of care for this patient.

    b. What teaching is appropriate for this patient?

34. A 60-year-old male utility worker was admitted to the emergency department with symptoms of hyponatremia following an 8-hour workday. The environmental temperature averaged 75 degrees.

    a. What additional assessment data are important for the nurse to gather?

    b. What nursing interventions would be appropriate to assist this patient in avoiding hyponatremia in the future?

CHAPTER 25

DRUGS FOR HYPERTENSION

FILL IN THE BLANK

From the textbook, find the correct word(s) to complete the statement(s).

1. High blood pressure that has no identifiable cause is called _____ _____.

2. Angiotensin II raises blood pressure by _____ _____ _____.

3. Calcium channel blockers cause the smooth muscle in arterioles to_____, thus_____ blood pressure.

4. ACE inhibitors such as captopril (Capoten) reduce blood pressure by lowering levels of _____ and _____.

5. _____ _____ is a condition that occurs when the heart rate increases due to the rapid fall in blood pressure created by a drug.

6. The side effects of adrenergic blockers are generally quite predictable, since they are usually extensions of the _____ _____ _____ response.

7. _____ act on the kidney and are often first-line medications for the treatment of hypertension.

Adams/Holland, *Student Workbook and Resource Guide for Pharmacology for Nurses* 4th Edition
© 2014 by Pearson Education, Inc.

MATCHING

For questions 8 through 16, match the drug in column I with its pharmacologic classification in column II.

Column I	Column II
8. _____ clonidine (Catapres)	a. diuretic
9. _____ captopril (Capoten)	b. calcium channel blocker
10. _____ spironolactone (Aldactone)	c. ACE inhibitor or angiotensin receptor blocker
11. _____ losartan (Cozaar)	d. beta$_1$ blocker
12. _____ verapamil (Calan)	e. alpha$_1$ blocker
13. _____ lisinopril (Prinivil)	f. centrally acting alpha$_2$ agonist
14. _____ hydralazine (Apresoline)	g. direct vasodilator
15. _____ metoprolol (Toprol)	
16. _____ hydrochlorothiazide (Microzide)	

MULTIPLE CHOICE

17. Which of the following lowers blood pressure primarily by increasing the renal excretion of sodium and water?

 a. Doxazosin (Cardura)

 b. Furosemide (Lasix)

 c. Verapamil (Calan)

 d. Quinapril (Accupril)

18. Which of the following is a cardioselective beta$_1$ blocker?

 a. Propranolol (Inderal)

 b. Doxazosin (Cardura)

 c. Ipratropium (Atrovent)

 d. Atenolol (Tenormin)

19. The nurse takes a patient's blood pressure at 157/93 mmHg. In an adult patient this level is considered:

 a. normal.

 b. prehypertensive.

 c. hypertension, stage 1.

 d. hypertension, stage 2.

20. Which of the following is NOT a primary factor responsible for blood pressure?

 a. Venous pressure

 b. Cardiac output

 c. Resistance of the small arteries

 d. Blood volume

21. During antihypertensive therapy, it is common practice to implement:

    a. two or more drugs from the same class.

    b. two or more drugs from different classes.

    c. one drug during weeks 1 to 3, then a new drug starting in week 4.

    d. one week of drug therapy alternating with 1 week of no drug administration.

22. When developing a plan of care, the nurse should know that which drug class is NOT commonly used to treat hypertension?

    a. Calcium channel blockers

    b. Angiotensin-converting enzyme inhibitors

    c. Direct-acting vasodilators

    d. Sodium channel blockers

23. Which of the following classes are preferred drugs for treating mild to moderate hypertension because they act on the kidney tubule to block reabsorption of sodium?

    a. Diuretics

    b. Calcium channel blockers

    c. Direct vasodilators

    d. Alpha blockers

24. The nurse should carefully monitor for hyperkalemia when patients are taking which class of drug?

    a. Diuretics

    b. Calcium channel blockers

    c. Direct vasodilators

    d. Alpha blockers

25. Calcium channel blockers used for hypertension act by blocking calcium ion channels in which of the following?

    a. Skeletal muscle

    b. Vascular smooth muscle

    c. Central nervous system

    d. Kidney

26. Which drug class will inhibit the secretion of aldosterone?

    a. Diuretics

    b. Calcium channel blockers

    c. ACE inhibitors

    d. Alpha blockers

27. Which of the following classes of autonomic drugs is used to treat hypertension?

    a. Sympathomimetics

    b. Alpha adrenergic agonists

    c. Selective $beta_2$ blockers

    d. Parasympathomimetics

28. The nurse carefully monitors for bradycardia in patients taking which of the following?

    a. Selective $beta_1$ blockers

    b. Calcium channel blockers

    c. ACE inhibitors

    d. Alpha blockers

29. The nurse is treating a patient who is having a hypertensive emergency. The nurse should know that which of the following drugs is given intravenously to lower high blood pressure within minutes?

    a. Hydralazine (Apresoline)

    b. Nitroprusside (Nitropress)

    c. Doxazosin (Cardura)

    d. Prazosin (Minipress)

30. In response to falling blood pressure, what do the kidneys release?

    a. Renin

    b. Aldosterone

    c. Angiotensin

    d. Potassium

31. In asthmatic patients, the nurse should monitor carefully for signs and symptoms of bronchoconstriction when using which class of antihypertensives?

    a. Alpha blockers

    b. Calcium channel blockers

    c. ACE inhibitors

    d. Beta blockers

MAKING CONNECTIONS

32. The nurse assesses for rhabdomyolysis in patients receiving:

    a. statins

    b. opioids

    c. selective serotoxin reuptake inhibitors (SSRIs)

    d. fibric acid agents

33. Which of the following routes for hydromorphone should be used to achieve the most rapid onset of action?

   a. PO 8.0 mg

   b. SC 1.5 mg

   c. IV 0.80 mg

   d. Rectal 3.0 mg

34. For hypertension, the nurse administers an average daily dose of 5 mg for enalapril and 10.0 mg for fosinopril. From this information, what may the nurse correctly conclude?

   a. Enalapril is twice as efficacious as fosinopril.

   b. Enalapril will likely produce fewer side effects than fosinopril.

   c. Enalapril is more potent than fosinopril.

   d. The onset of action for fosinopril will be longer than that of enalapril.

35. Atropine is a prototype for which drug class?

   a. Sympathomimetics

   b. Beta-adrenergic blockers

   c. Parasympathomimetics

   d. Cholinergic blockers

36. Which of the following drugs is often combined in cartridges with local anesthetics?

   a. Epinephrine

   b. Atropine

   c. Heparin

   d. Acetaminophen

CALCULATIONS

37. Furosemide 15 mg is ordered. The bottle reads: 20 mg/2 mL. How much furosemide will the nurse draw up in the syringe?

38. A cardiac patient has Cardizem 60 mg qid ordered. How many tablets will the nurse administer for each dose if the bottle reads diltiazem HCl (Cardizem) 120 mg/tablet?

CASE STUDY APPLICATIONS

39. A 50-year-old male has presented with a blood pressure of 170/100 mmHg the last two visits to his health care provider. Hydrochlorothiazide (Microzide) was prescribed for him about 1 year ago. Other than some anxiety, he offers no complaints and other vital signs are normal. His blood lipids are elevated, he is 20 lb overweight, and he smokes a pack of cigarettes a day; otherwise, he appears healthy.

   a. What assessment data help the nurse understand the contributing factors for this patient's hypertension?

   b. The nurse suspects that this patient has not been taking his medication. What nursing diagnoses would the nurse identify? What outcomes would the nurse select for the diagnoses?

   c. Assuming this patient has been taking his hydrochlorothiazide, what is the next logical pharmacologic option for him?

40. A 75-year-old female has been taking enalapril (Vasotec) and chlorothiazide for hypertension for the past 2 years. She is very compliant, taking walks daily, watching her salt intake, and eating plenty of potassium-rich foods such as bananas. Two weeks ago, her health care provider increased her dose of enalapril and switched her to spironolactone instead of chlorothiazide. She is now in the office complaining that she gets dizzy and falls over every morning when she gets out of bed, and that she feels like her heart is racing when she walks. Although her blood pressure is normal, she wants to be switched back to her previous medications.

a. What assessment data lead the nurse to understand the potential cause of her dizziness? What teaching might be done to help solve this problem?

b. An ECG on this patient is normal. Is there anything in her history that might be responsible for her heart complaints? What assessment information would help the nurse define her problem?

c. Is it necessary to change this patient's medication, or is it possible that her complaints could be resolved through patient teaching?

CHAPTER 26

DRUGS FOR HEART FAILURE

FILL IN THE BLANK

From the textbook, find the correct word(s) to complete the statement(s).

1. As more stretch is applied to myocardial fibers, they will contract with greater force. This is known as the _____ law.

2. As a general rule, if the heart rate is less than _____ beats per minute, digoxin (Lanoxin) should not be administered.

3. The two most important variables that affect cardiac output are _____ and _____.

4. When a medication has a positive inotropic effect, it has the ability to _____ the _____ of the myocardial contraction.

5. Cardiac glycosides cause the heart to beat more _____ and more _____.

6. If a patient has taken an overdose of digoxin, the health care provider will administer _____ _____ _____ to treat this life-threatening condition.

7. Blocking the enzyme phosphodiesterase has the effect of increasing the amount of _____ ion available for myocardial contraction.

Adams/Holland, *Student Workbook and Resource Guide for Pharmacology for Nurses* 4th Edition
© 2014 by Pearson Education, Inc.

MATCHING

For questions 8 through 16, match the drug in column I with its classification in column II.

Column I	Column II
8. _____ lisinopril (Prinivil)	a. diuretic
9. _____ hydralazine (Apresoline)	b. cardiac glycoside
10. _____ carvedilol (Coreg)	c. ACE inhibitor
11. _____ hydrochlorothiazide (Microzide)	d. beta blocker
12. _____ milrinone (Primacor)	e. direct vasodilator
13. _____ quinapril (Accupril)	f. phosphodiesterase inhibitor
14. _____ metoprolol (Toprol XL)	
15. _____ enalapril (Vasotec)	
16. _____ isosorbide dinitrate (Isordil)	

MULTIPLE CHOICE

17. The primary action of digoxin (Lanoxin) that makes it very effective at treating heart failure is its ability to:

    a. dilate the coronary arteries.

    b. increase impulse conduction across the myocardium.

    c. decrease blood pressure.

    d. increase cardiac contractility/output.

18. Blood electrolyte levels are critical to safe digoxin therapy. The nurse must carefully monitor for which of the following, which significantly reduces the effectiveness of digoxin?

    a. Hypokalemia

    b. Hyperkalemia

    c. Hypocalcemia

    d. Hypercalcemia

19. What is the best definition of heart failure?

    a. Enlargement of the heart

    b. Inability of the heart to beat in a coordinated manner

    c. Inability of the ventricles to pump sufficient blood

    d. Congestion in the lungs caused by damage to the myocardium

20. What is the amount of blood pumped by each ventricle per minute called?

    a. Preload

    b. Afterload

    c. Stroke volume

    d. Cardiac output

21. What is the correct definition of preload?

    a. Amount of blood pumped by each ventricle per minute

    b. Degree to which the heart fibers are stretched just prior to contraction

    c. Pressure in the aorta that must be overcome for blood to be ejected from the heart

    d. Ability to increase the strength of contraction

22. When monitoring patients on cardiac glycosides, the nurse knows that these drugs help the heart to beat more forcefully and:

    a. with a faster heart rate.

    b. with a slower heart rate.

    c. do not affect cardiac output.

    d. with a diminished cardiac output.

23. Digoxin (Lanoxin) acts by which of the following?

    a. Blocking beta-adrenergic receptors in the heart

    b. Stimulating beta-adrenergic receptors in the heart

    c. Inhibiting Na^+-K^+ ATPase

    d. Stimulating Na^+-K^+ ATPase

24. The nurse should carefully monitor for which of the following adverse effects in a patient taking digoxin for heart failure?

    a. Rhythm abnormalities

    b. Increased cardiac output

    c. Increased urine production

    d. Decreased blood pressure

25. Which drug class has largely replaced the cardiac glycosides as first-line drugs in the therapy of heart failure?

    a. Direct vasodilators

    b. ACE inhibitors

    c. Phosphodiesterase inhibitors

    d. Beta-adrenergic blockers

26. The primary action of the ACE inhibitors that benefits a patient with heart failure is a decrease in:

    a. peripheral resistance/blood pressure.

    b. cardiac output.

    c. heart rate.

    d. urine output.

27. By what mechanism does isosorbide dinitrate (Isordil) benefit patients with heart failure?

    a. Lowering arterial blood pressure

    b. Increasing urine output

    c. Reducing venous return, causing a decrease in cardiac workload

    d. Slowing the heart rate, causing a reduction in cardiac workload

28. In addition to heart failure, what is hydralazine (Apresoline) also prescribed for?

    a. Coagulation disorders

    b. Hypertension

    c. Stroke

    d. Glaucoma

29. In addition to heart failure, what are diuretics also commonly prescribed for?

    a. Minor depression

    b. Coagulation disorders

    c. Hypertension

    d. Dysrhythmias

30. By what mechanism do diuretics such as furosemide (Lasix) improve the symptoms of heart failure?

    a. Blocking beta-adrenergic receptors

    b. Causing the heart to beat with more strength

    c. Reducing fluid/plasma volume

    d. Slowing heart rate, thus reducing cardiac workload

31. The nurse must carefully monitor for which of the following serious adverse effects of furosemide (Lasix) therapy?

    a. Electrolyte imbalances

    b. Dysrhythmias

    c. Reflex tachycardia

    d. Hypertension

32. What is the primary use of the phosphodiesterase inhibitors in heart failure patients?

    a. Cause a rapid reduction in fluid/plasma volume

    b. Cause the heart to beat faster

    c. Rapidly lower blood pressure

    d. Increase the force of contraction and increase cardiac output

33. How do beta-adrenergic blockers such as carvedilol (Coreg) improve symptoms of heart failure?

    a. Increase heart rate

    b. Decrease heart rate

    c. Cause the heart to contract with more force

    d. Lower blood pressure and reduce cardiac workload

MAKING CONNECTIONS

34. Which of the following drugs acts by inhibiting aldosterone?

    a. Spironolactone (Aldactone)

    b. Hydralazine (Apresoline)

    c. Metoprolol (Toprol XL)

    d. Furosemide (Lasix)

35. The nurse should teach patients to eat plenty of bananas during pharmacotherapy with thiazide diuretics, to obtain an adequate amount of which of the following?

    a. Selenium

    b. Calcium

    c. Potassium

    d. Chloride

36. The nurse is asked to administer carvedilol 6.25 mg bid. What does the term *bid* mean?

    a. Twice a week

    b. Twice a day

    c. Before bedtime

    d. Before breakfast

37. Which of the following drug classes does NOT have significant potential for abuse by patients?

    a. Barbiturates

    b. Benzodiazepines

    c. Opioids

    d. Anticholinergics

38. Which drug class may be used to dry secretions, treat asthma, and prevent motion sickness?

    a. Anticholinergics

    b. Cholinergics

    c. Parasympathomimetics

    d. Alpha blockers

CALCULATIONS

39. A solution of amrinone lactate 100 mg in 40 mL NS is ordered to infuse at 5 mcg/kg/min for a patient weighing 75 kg. What is the milliliter per hour flow rate?

40. A physician orders furosemide 40 mg IV push. The bottle label reads: furosemide 20 mg/2 mL. How many milliliters will the nurse give?

CASE STUDY APPLICATIONS

41. Drugs can affect the heart in a number of ways. It is essential that the nurse understand the underlying cardiac pathophysiology in order to understand drug action.

    a. Explain the difference between an inotropic effect and a chronotropic effect.

    b. Give examples of pharmacologic classes of drugs that affect each.

    c. In general, is it more desirable to give a drug with a positive inotropic effect or a positive chronotropic effect when treating chronic heart failure? Explain the answer.

42. A male has just been diagnosed with early heart failure and his health care provider has prescribed hydrochlorothiazide (Microzide), atorvastatin (Lipitor), and lisinopril (Prinivil). His blood pressure is slightly elevated, his blood cholesterol is marginally high, and he has stenosis of the mitral valve that seems to be worsening. Although the patient is not an athletic person, he likes to take long walks after dinner. He confides that at his age of 60 he has no intention of taking any of the medications, but intends to try Chinese herbal therapy.

    a. The nurse is developing a teaching plan for this patient. The nurse wants to explain the rationale for each of the patient's medications. What information will the nurse include in the teaching plan?

    b. How does the nurse assess the patient's need for alternative therapy, and what is the best response to his concern about prescription drugs?

    c. Knowing that health promotion is an essential nursing action, what lifestyle changes would the nurse suggest to this patient to improve his cardiac health?

43. An elderly female patient is transferred from a rehabilitation center to an acute care setting with a diagnosis of heart failure and the following vital signs: BP 120/90, pulse 108/min, and labored respiration 32/min. Assessment of breath sounds reveals coarse rhonchi and wheezing on inspiration and expiration. A 10-lb weight gain has been observed over a 3-day period. The care plan includes digoxin 0.5 mg IV STAT to be repeated in 4 hours and then an oral dose of 0.25 mg/day.

    a. What assessment data support the diagnosis of heart failure?

    b. Why would the care plan include a STAT dose of digoxin with a dose repeating in 4 hours and then a lower daily dose?

    c. What other bodily system must the nurse pay close attention to in the assessment of this patient with heart failure?

CHAPTER 27

DRUGS FOR ANGINA PECTORIS AND MYOCARDIAL INFARCTION

FILL IN THE BLANK

From the textbook, find the correct word(s) to complete the statement(s).

1. Acute chest pain on physical exertion or emotional stress is a characteristic symptom of _____ _____.

2. Atherosclerosis is due to a buildup of fatty, fibrous material called _____ in the walls of arteries.

3. The type of angina pectoris that is predictable in its frequency and duration is called _____ angina.

4. Drug therapy of stable angina usually begins with _____ _____.

5. Long-acting nitrates are often delivered through a _____ _____ to decrease the frequency and severity of anginal episodes.

6. After a clot in the coronary artery has been successfully dissolved, therapy with _____ is often initiated to prevent the formation of additional thrombi.

MATCHING

For questions 7 through 13, match the drug in column I with its classification in column II.

Column I	Column II
7. _____ diltiazem (Cardizem)	a. organic nitrate
8. _____ isosorbide dinitrate (Dilatrate)	b. beta blocker
9. _____ metoprolol (Lopressor)	c. calcium channel blocker
10. _____ atenolol (Tenormin)	d. ACE inhibitor
11. _____ nifedipine (Procardia)	
12. _____ nitroglycerin (Nitrostat)	
13. _____ amlodipine (Norvasc)	

MULTIPLE CHOICE

14. Which of the following drug classes is prescribed for patients with angina pectoris?

    a. Calcium channel blockers

    b. ACE inhibitors

    c. HMG-CoA reductase inhibitors

    d. Cardiac glycosides

15. Which of the following best explains the mechanism by which organic nitrates terminate variant angina?

    a. Direct vasodilation of coronary arteries

    b. Slowing heart rate

    c. Stronger force of myocardial contraction

    d. Dilation of peripheral veins, reducing preload

16. What is the condition of having a reduced blood supply to myocardial cells called?

    a. Myocardial infarction

    b. Angina pectoris

    c. Myocardial ischemia

    d. Stroke

17. In assessing a patient with chest pain, the nurse knows that angina is most often preceded by which of the following?

    a. An aura

    b. Physical exertion or emotional excitement

    c. A sensation that the heart has skipped a beat

    d. Severe pain down the left arm

18. The pharmacologic goals for the treatment of angina are usually achieved by which of the following?

    a. Reducing cardiac workload

    b. Increasing heart rate

    c. Increasing force of myocardial contraction

    d. Increasing amount of blood entering the heart

19. By causing venodilation, nitrates reduce the amount of blood returning to the heart, thus decreasing which of the following?

    a. Heart rate

    b. Conduction velocity

    c. Ischemia

    d. Cardiac output

20. In addition to causing venodilation, organic nitrates also have the ability to:

    a. inhibit alpha$_1$-adrenergic receptors in arterioles.

    b. dilate the coronary arteries.

    c. terminate dysrhythmias.

    d. remove plaque from coronary arteries.

21. Organic nitrates are classified based on whether they are:

    a. parenteral or oral.

    b. high or low potency.

    c. short or long acting.

    d. sedating or nonsedating.

22. Which drug would the nurse administer sublingually to rapidly terminate angina pain?

    a. Atenolol (Tenormin)

    b. Diltiazem (Cardizem)

    c. Nitroglycerin (Nitro-Bid)

    d. Aspirin (Bayer)

23. A patient is receiving nitroglycerin (Nitro-Bid). The nurse should monitor for the most common adverse effect, which is:

    a. headache.

    b. drowsiness.

    c. nausea/vomiting.

    d. hypotension.

24. What is the primary mechanism by which beta-adrenergic blockers decrease the frequency of angina attacks?

    a. Dilating the coronary arteries

    b. Increasing the heart rate

    c. Increasing the strength of contraction of the myocardium

    d. Reducing cardiac workload

25. Which of the following is true regarding the effect of atenolol (Tenormin) on the heart?

    a. Selective $beta_1$ receptor blocker

    b. Nonselective $beta_1$ and $beta_2$ blocker

    c. Selective $beta_2$ receptor blocker

    d. Has no effect on beta receptors

26. What is the primary mechanism by which calcium channel blockers decrease the frequency of angina attacks?

    a. Slow conduction through the SA node

    b. Increase the heart rate

    c. Increase the strength of contraction of the myocardium

    d. Reduce cardiac workload

27. Calcium channel blockers are useful in treating variant angina because they do which of the following?

    a. Lower blood pressure

    b. Slow the heart rate

    c. Slow conduction across the myocardium

    d. Relax arterial smooth muscle in the coronary arteries

28. Which of the following drugs has the ability to inhibit the transport of calcium ions into myocardial cells, and the ability to relax both coronary and peripheral blood vessels?

    a. Atenolol (Tenormin)

    b. Diltiazem (Cardizem)

    c. Nitroglycerin (Nitro-Bid)

    d. Reteplase (Retavase)

29. Which of the following is NOT a goal for the pharmacotherapy of acute myocardial infarction (MI)?

    a. Restore blood supply to the damaged myocardium as quickly as possible

    b. Increase myocardial oxygen demand with organic nitrates or beta blockers

    c. Prevent associated dysrhythmias with antidysrhythmic medications

    d. Reduce post-MI mortality with aspirin and ACE inhibitors

30. In treating a patient with a recent MI, the nurse knows that the function of thrombolytic therapy is to do which of the following?

    a. Restore blood supply to the damaged myocardium

    b. Decrease myocardial oxygen demand

    c. Control dysrhythmias

    d. Reduce acute pain associated with MI

31. The nurse administering a thrombolytic drug should monitor for which of the following primary adverse effects?

    a. Hypertension

    b. Prolonged prothrombin time

    c. Excessive bleeding

    d. Dysrhythmia

32. The nurse should know that reteplase (Retavase) is most effective if given within what time frame after the onset of MI symptoms?

    a. 30 minutes

    b. 1 hour

    c. 6 hours

    d. 12 hours

33. Following an acute MI, metoprolol (Lopressor) is infused slowly until which of the following occurs?

    a. The clot is dissolved.

    b. Blood pressure falls to 100/70 mmHg.

    c. A target heart rate of 60 to 90 beats per minute is reached.

    d. The pain is relieved.

34. Unless contraindicated, 160 to 324 mg of aspirin is administered as soon as possible following a suspected MI in order to:

    a. restore blood supply to the damaged myocardium.

    b. decrease myocardial oxygen demand.

    c. reduce post-MI mortality.

    d. reduce acute pain associated with MI.

35. Why is captopril (Capoten) prescribed for patients who have experienced a recent myocardial infarction (MI)?

    a. To restore blood supply to the damaged myocardium

    b. To increase myocardial oxygen demand

    c. To reduce post-MI mortality

    d. To reduce acute pain associated with MI

36. Why does the nurse administer opioids such as morphine sulfate following an MI?

    a. To restore blood supply to the damaged myocardium

    b. To decrease myocardial oxygen demand

    c. To reduce post-MI mortality

    d. To reduce acute pain associated with MI

MAKING CONNECTIONS

37. In addition to angina, the nurse may administer organic nitrates to treat which of the following?

    a. Dysrhythmias

    b. Coagulation disorders

    c. Hypertension

    d. Heart failure

38. What is the classification of nitrous oxide?

    a. IV anesthetic

    b. Gas

    c. Volatile agent

    d. Local anesthetic

39. Extrapyramidal adverse effects are observed during therapy with which drug group?

    a. Antianxiety drugs

    b. Antipsychotics

    c. Antiepilepsy drugs

    d. Opioids

40. A patient taking lithium (Eskalith) is likely being treated for which of the following conditions?

    a. Bipolar disorder

    b. Schizophrenia

    c. Attention deficit/hyperactivity disorder

    d. Mild to moderate pain

41. Which of the following blocks impulses from the parasympathetic nervous system?

    a. Sympathomimetic

    b. Beta-adrenergic blocker

    c. Cholinergic blocker

    d. Calcium channel blocker

CALCULATIONS

42. A nitroglycerin solution of 50 mg/250 mL D5W is infused at 15 gtt/min. The IV set calibration is 60 gtt/mL. How many micrograms per minute are infused?

43. A patient has an IV drip of Cardizem 125 mg/100 mL D5W. The health care provider orders Cardizem 10 mg/h. How many drops per minute will the nurse give if a microdrip is used?

CASE STUDY APPLICATIONS

44. A 70-year-old, 280-lb man is admitted through the emergency department for a possible stroke. His physical exam reveals he is alert, with a pulse of 76 regular, BP 190/110 mmHg, respirations 24/min, and slurred speech. He has significant weakness in the left arm, left hand, and left leg. A computed tomography (CT) scan confirms a recent stroke. His social history includes occasional alcohol use and two packs per day tobacco use for 50 years. He is a retired accountant, is married, and has seven adult children and 16 grandchildren. During hospitalization, he was given reteplase (Retavase), furosemide (Lasix), and heparin. He was discharged with the following medications: hydrochlorothiazide (Microzide), diltiazem (Cardizem), and warfarin (Coumadin).

    a. After analysis of the admission data, what risk factors have likely contributed to this patient's stroke?

    b. After the nurse reviews the medications, what rationale supports the delivery of Retavase, Lasix, and heparin?

    c. The nurse is preparing to begin discharge teaching. What rationale will the nurse give this patient for the use of Microzide, Coumadin, and Cardizem?

45. A 72-year-old woman who has been treated several times for chronic heart failure, hypertension, and angina presents with a complaint of frequent and intense anginal pain. She has chest pain with minor exertion and headaches with the use of prn nitroglycerin. Her current medications are isosorbide dinitrate, nitroglycerin, atenolol (Tenormin), and amlodipine (Norvasc). Physical exam reveals the patient is alert, oriented, BP 164/92 mmHg, pulse 66 regular, respirations 28, skin cool, strength equal in all extremities, edema in lower extremities, and a weight gain of 7 lb in 3 weeks.

    a. After analysis of this patient situation, what nursing diagnoses will the nurse identify?

    b. What assessment data support the possibility of side effects from Norvasc?

    c. Why are the nitrates not relieving the patient's pain?

CHAPTER 28

DRUGS FOR SHOCK

FILL IN THE BLANK

From the textbook, find the correct word(s) to complete the statement(s).

1. In the early stages of shock, the body compensates for the fall in blood pressure by increasing the activity of the _____ nervous system.

2. Norepinephrine acts directly on _____ adrenergic receptors to constrict arteries and raise blood pressure.

3. At low doses dopamine selectively stimulates _____ receptors, whereas at higher doses it stimulates _____ receptors.

4. Dopamine is used to increase the force of the myocardial contraction by stimulating _____ receptors.

5. The first goal in the treatment of shock is to provide _____ _____ _____.

6. _____ _____ may be indicated for the treatment of acute, massive blood loss (more than 30% of the total volume).

7. The major adverse outcome when using a colloid to treat shock is _____ _____.

8. When given in large doses, colloids such as hetastarch can increase laboratory values of _____, _____, and _____ _____.

Adams/Holland, *Student Workbook and Resource Guide for Pharmacology for Nurses* 4th Edition

MATCHING

For questions 9 through 15, match the drug in column I with its primary class in column II.

Column I	Column II
9. _____ norepinephrine	a. vasoconstrictor or inotropic
10. _____ digoxin (Lanoxin)	b. colloid
11. _____ phenylephrine	c. crystalloid
12. _____ dextran 40	d. blood product
13. _____ dopamine (Dopastat)	
14. _____ platelets	
15. _____ normal saline	

MULTIPLE CHOICE

16. The nurse is administering epinephrine: 0.25 mL of 1:1,000, every 10 min. Which of the following should the nurse monitor to prevent overdose from the drug?

    a. Hypoglycemia

    b. Hypertension

    c. Bronchospasm

    d. Diarrhea

17. Shock is a condition characterized by which of the following?

    a. Extremely high blood pressure

    b. Abnormal cardiac rhythm

    c. Vital tissues not receiving enough blood to function properly

    d. The heart not pumping with sufficient contractility

18. Which of the following is NOT a common sign or symptom of shock?

    a. Feeling weak, with nonspecific symptoms

    b. Restlessness, anxiety, confusion, lack of interest

    c. Thirst

    d. Hypertension

19. A weak or unresponsive patient with obvious trauma or bleeding to a limb might be experiencing what type of shock?

    a. Hypovolemic

    b. Neurogenic

    c. Cardiogenic

    d. Anaphylactic

20. In many types of shock, what is the most serious medical challenge facing the patient?

    a. Heart failure

    b. Brain damage

    c. Hypotension

    d. MI

21. What is the purpose of administering vasoconstrictors to a patient with shock?

    a. To prevent dysrhythmias

    b. To stabilize blood pressure

    c. To prevent postshock mortality

    d. To prevent blood pressure from rising to harmful levels

22. Most of the drugs used to raise blood pressure in patients with shock:

    a. are CNS stimulants.

    b. are CNS depressants.

    c. activate the parasympathetic nervous system.

    d. activate the sympathetic nervous system.

23. Norepinephrine activates which adrenergic receptors?

    a. Alpha

    b. $Beta_1$

    c. Both alpha and $beta_1$

    d. Neither alpha nor $beta_1$

24. In addition to its use in shock, norepinephrine is also of value in treating which of the following?

    a. Cardiac arrest

    b. Hypertension

    c. Dysrhythmias

    d. Strokes

25. The primary use of cardiotonic drugs in the treatment of shock is to increase which of the following?

    a. Blood pressure

    b. Force of myocardial contraction

    c. Heart rate

    d. Conduction velocity across the myocardium

26. The nurse is ready to administer dobutamine (Dobutrex) 2.5 mcg/kg for 5 min. The nurse should know that this drug belongs to which of the following drug classes?

    a. Selective beta$_1$ blocker

    b. Cholinergic blocker

    c. Cardiac glycoside

    d. Beta$_1$-adrenergic agonist

27. Which of the following drug classes consists of large molecules that draw water molecules away from cells and tissues into blood vessels?

    a. Crystalloids

    b. Hypovolemics

    c. Inotropics

    d. Colloids

MAKING CONNECTIONS

28. Which of the following is an expected effect when the nurse administers a beta-adrenergic blocker?

    a. Increased heart rate

    b. Lowered blood pressure

    c. Dilation of bronchial smooth muscle

    d. Increased myocardial contractility

29. Which of the following is a cholinergic blocker?

    a. Metoprolol (Lopressor)

    b. Succinylcholine (Anectine)

    c. Neostigmine (Prostigmin)

    d. Atropine sulfate

30. Which of the following is NOT classified as an NSAID?

    a. Acetaminophen

    b. Aspirin

    c. Celecoxib (Celebrex)

    d. Ibuprofen

31. Antiplatelet agents are primarily prescribed to do which of the following?

    a. Lower blood cholesterol

    b. Dissolve thrombi

    c. Prevent thrombi from forming

    d. Prevent migraines

32. Most barbiturate use in children is limited to treating which of the following?

    a. Sleep disorders

    b. Seizure disorders

    c. Depression

    d. Anxiety

CALCULATIONS

33. Dopamine has been ordered at 4 mcg/kg/min using a 400 mg/250 mL D5W solution. The patient weighs 92.4 kg. Calculate the dosage-per-minute and milliliter-per-hour flow rate.

34. Dobutrex 5 mcg/kg/min has been ordered using a 500 mg/250 mL D5W solution. The patient weighs 99.4 kg. Calculate the milliliter-per-hour flow rate.

CASE STUDY APPLICATIONS

35. Paramedics arrive at the scene of an automobile accident and discover a 35-year-old victim who is wandering around the scene confused. The patient has several superficial wounds that are bleeding, although the amount of blood does not appear to be great. Initial vital signs show slightly elevated blood pressure and weak pulse. The paramedics treat the wounds, administer oxygen, and keep the patient warm and lying on a stretcher while they treat other injured people at the scene. Twenty minutes later, the patient is unresponsive with a blood pressure of 70/40 and no identifiable pulse. EKG reveals a ventricular dysrhythmia that appears to be quickly worsening. The paramedics immediately administer the following drugs:

    dextran 70 (Macrodex)

    norepinephrine (Levophed)

    dobutamine (Dobutrex)

    lidocaine (Xylocaine)

    a. What assessment data support a diagnosis of hypovolemic shock?

    b. What nursing diagnosis would be most appropriate at the scene of this accident?

    c. What is the rationale for each drug and how will the nurse evaluate effectiveness?

36. At the same auto accident described in the previous question, paramedics find an elderly patient who has a closed head injury. The patient is unconscious and has no bleeding evident. Vital signs show slow respirations, very low pulse rate, and a blood pressure of 94/52. Pupils are unresponsive to light.

    a. What type of shock is this patient most likely experiencing? List all assessment data that lead to this conclusion.

    b. What drugs would the nurse expect to administer to reverse the symptoms of shock?

    c. What data would lead the nurse to evaluate this case as being a successfully treated case of neurogenic shock?

CHAPTER 29

DRUGS FOR DYSRHYTHMIAS

FILL IN THE BLANK

From the textbook, find the correct word(s) to complete the statement(s).

1. After the action potential has passed and the myocardial cell is in a depolarized state, repolarization depends on removal of _____ ion from the cell.

2. Calcium channel blockers are only effective against _____ dysrhythmias.

3. Severe dysrhythmias may result in _____ _____.

4. The most common type of dysrhythmia is _____ _____.

5. Procainamide and quinidine act by blocking _____ _____.

6. Beta blockers will _____ the heart rate and _____ the velocity of the action potential traveling through the atrioventricular node.

7. Label the parts of the conduction pathway and the events of the ECG in Figure 29–1.

   A. _____   E. _____

   B. _____   F. _____

   C. _____   G. _____

   D. _____   H. _____

Adams/Holland, *Student Workbook and Resource Guide for Pharmacology for Nurses* 4th Edition
© 2014 by Pearson Education, Inc.

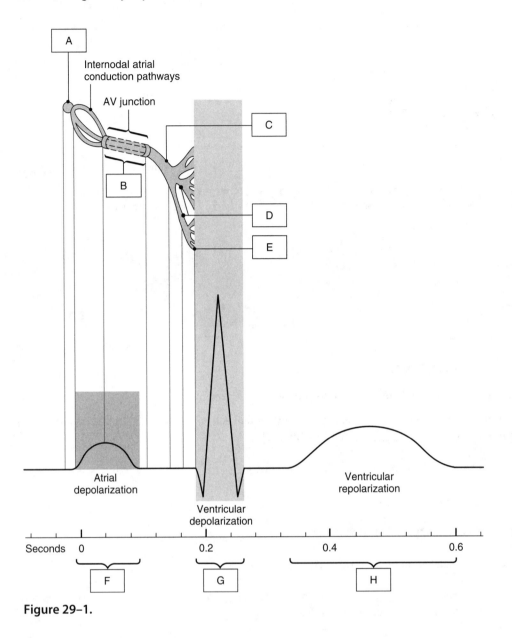

Figure 29–1.

MATCHING

For questions 8 through 16, match the drug in column I with its classification in column II.

Column I	Column II
8. _____ quinidine gluconate	a. sodium channel blocker
9. _____ amiodarone (Cordarone)	b. potassium channel blocker
10. _____ diltiazem (Cardizem)	c. beta-adrenergic blocker
11. _____ verapamil (Calan)	d. calcium channel blocker
12. _____ phenytoin (Dilantin)	e. miscellaneous (none of the above)
13. _____ propranolol (Inderal)	
14. _____ lidocaine (Xylocaine)	
15. _____ procainamide	
16. _____ adenosine (Adenocard)	

MULTIPLE CHOICE

17. Which of the following best describes dysrhythmias?

    a. Abnormalities of electrical conduction in the heart

    b. Diminished cardiac output

    c. Narrowing of the coronary arteries

    d. High blood pressure

18. Which of the following is NOT a type of dysrhythmia?

    a. Atrial tachycardia

    b. Ventricular flutter

    c. Sinus bradycardia

    d. Premature subventricular contractions

19. Where does cardiac conduction begin?

    a. Atrioventricular bundle

    b. Atrioventricular (AV) node

    c. Sinoatrial (SA) node

    d. Purkinje fibers

20. Under resting conditions, a new action potential crosses the myocardium approximately how many times every minute?

    a. 60

    b. 75

    c. 85

    d. 110

21. In most myocardial cells and in neurons, an action potential begins when channels located in the plasma membrane open and _____ rushes into the cell, producing a rapid depolarization.

    a. calcium

    b. phosphate

    c. potassium

    d. sodium

22. Which of the following is NOT a class of drugs used to treat dysrhythmias?

    a. Sodium channel blockers

    b. Alpha-adrenergic blockers

    c. Potassium channel blockers

    d. Calcium channel blockers

23. Which of the following is the basic mechanism by which nearly all antidysrhythmic drugs terminate or prevent abnormal cardiac rhythms?

    a. They increase heart rate until cardiac rhythm returns to normal.

    b. They dilate coronary arteries so that more blood gets to the myocardium.

    c. They slow the impulse conduction velocity until cardiac rhythm returns to normal.

    d. They lower the blood pressure so the heart has less workload.

24. A blockade of sodium channels in myocardial cells will do which of the following?

    a. Slow the spread of impulse conduction across the myocardium

    b. Speed the spread of impulse conduction across the myocardium

    c. Stop the spread of impulse conduction across the myocardium

    d. Worsen a dysrhythmia

25. The physician orders 50 mg lidocaine for a patient with a dysrhythmia. The nurse will administer this drug by the _____ route to terminate _____ dysrhythmias.

    a. PO, ventricular

    b. PO, atrial

    c. IV, atrial

    d. IV, ventricular

26. Which antidysrhythmic drug acts by blocking beta-adrenergic receptors in the heart?

    a. Verapamil (Calan)

    b. Digoxin (Lanoxin)

    c. Amiodarone (Cordarone)

    d. Propranolol (Inderal)

27. Which of the following is a sodium channel blocker that is the oldest antidysrhythmic drug?

    a. Propranolol (Inderal)

    b. Amiodarone (Cordarone)

    c. Quinidine sulfate

    d. Verapamil (Calan)

28. The nurse is administering procainamide (Procanbid) for acute tachycardia. The nurse will assess for which unusual adverse drug effect that can affect 30% to 50% of patients?

    a. Stevens–Johnson syndrome

    b. Lupus

    c. Lymphoma

    d. Aplastic anemia

29. Beta-adrenergic blockers are used to treat a large number of cardiovascular diseases. Which of the following is NOT an indication for beta blocker therapy?

    a. Anticoagulant

    b. Hypertension

    c. Heart failure

    d. Dysrhythmias

30. How do beta-adrenergic blockers prevent dysrhythmias?

    a. They speed impulse conduction across the myocardium.

    b. They slow impulse conduction across the myocardium.

    c. They block calcium channels.

    d. They block sodium channels.

31. Propranolol (Inderal) is classified as which of the following?

    a. Nonselective alpha and beta blocker

    b. Nonselective beta blocker

    c. Selective $beta_1$ blocker

    d. Selective $beta_2$ blocker

32. Which of the following is NOT an expected adverse effect in a patient taking propranolol (Inderal)?

    a. Diminished sex drive

    b. Hypotension

    c. Bradycardia

    d. Tachycardia

33. How do potassium channel blockers prevent dysrhythmias?

    a. They block beta-adrenergic receptors in the myocardium.

    b. They reduce blood pressure.

    c. They interfere with calcium ion channels.

    d. They prolong the refractory period of the heart.

34. Which potassium channel blocker has become a preferred drug for the treatment of serious atrial dysrhythmias in patients with heart failure?

    a. Ibutilide (Corvert)

    b. Dofetilide (Tikosyn)

    c. Amiodarone (Cordarone)

    d. Sotalol (Betapace)

35. The nurse must carefully monitor for which serious adverse effect of amiodarone (Cordarone)?

    a. stroke

    b. pneumonia-like syndrome

    c. bleeding

    d. peptic ulcers

36. Blocking calcium ion channels has a number of effects on the heart and vascular system. These effects are most similar to which of the following?

    a. Sodium channel blockers

    b. Potassium channel blockers

    c. Beta-adrenergic blockers

    d. Cardiac glycosides

37. The nurse would administer which of the following antidysrhythmics IV to rapidly terminate serious atrial dysrhythmias?

    a. Adenosine (Adenocard)

    b. Amiodarone (Cordarone)

    c. Propranolol (Inderal)

    d. Verapamil (Calan)

MAKING CONNECTIONS

38. The main benefit of phosphodiesterase inhibitors is in the treatment of which of the following?

    a. Hypertension

    b. Coagulation disorders

    c. Heart failure

    d. Shock

39. Which of the following is the most widely used class of agents for the treatment of clinical depression?

    a. Barbiturates

    b. Na^+-K^+ ATPase inhibitors

    c. Benzodiazepines

    d. Selective serotonin reuptake inhibitors

40. A patient taking sumatriptan (Imitrex) likely suffers from which of the following?

    a. Sleep disorders

    b. Seizures

    c. Migraines

    d. Schizophrenia

41. What is GABA?

    a. A surgical procedure used to help patients who are psychotic

    b. A neurotransmitter

    c. A drug used to treat bipolar disorder

    d. A widely abused hallucinogen

CALCULATIONS

42. A solution of Cardizem 125 mg/100 mL D5W is to infuse at a rate of 20 mg/h. Calculate the milliliter-per-hour flow rate.

43. A patient with atrial fibrillation has amiodarone ordered at 0.5 mg/min. The concentration is amiodarone 900 mg in 250 mL D5W. How many milliliters per hour should the IV pump be programmed to deliver?

CASE STUDY APPLICATIONS

44. A 67-year-old woman is brought to the hospital by paramedics after collapsing on the street. She has a history of heart failure and has been taking digoxin (Lanoxin) and furosemide (Lasix). The emergency department (ED) physician determines that she is experiencing a myocardial infarction accompanied by severe tachycardia.

    a. The ED nurse should collect what assessment data before propranolol is started?

    b. The patient is also given amiodarone (Cordarone). What is the rationale for using this drug for this patient?

    c. The nurse should anticipate what adverse effects from the use of amiodarone and propranolol?

45. The nurse is working on a progressive care unit (PCU). The monitor technician tells the nurse that a patient, admitted for chest pain, is demonstrating paroxysmal supraventricular tachycardia. The nurse knows the patient has a prn order for verapamil (Calan) if supraventricular tachycardia occurs.

    a. What nursing assessment must the nurse make before administering Calan?

    b. If the patient will remain on Calan, what patient teaching must be done?

    c. What nursing diagnoses may be identified for this patient?

CHAPTER 30

DRUGS FOR COAGULATION DISORDERS

FILL IN THE BLANK

From the textbook, find the correct word(s) to complete the statement(s).

1. Identify steps in the coagulation cascade shown in Figure 30–1.

   A. _____

   B. _____

   C. _____

2. Hemostatic medications inhibit the conversion of plasminogen to _____.

3. _____ is a common herb that can interact with coagulation modifiers.

4. The _____ are a class of drugs that dissolve life-threatening clots.

5. _____ are drugs that stabilize clots and inhibit the removal of fibrin.

6. Two laboratory tests used to determine the effects of anticoagulants are _____ _____ and _____ _____ _____.

Adams/Holland, *Student Workbook and Resource Guide for Pharmacology for Nurses* 4th Edition
© 2014 by Pearson Education, Inc.

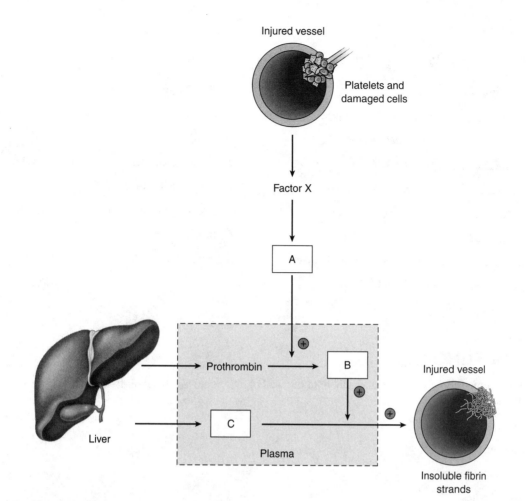

Figure 30–1.

MATCHING

For questions 7 through 14, match the drug in column I with its classification in column II.

Column I	Column II
7. _____ warfarin (Coumadin)	a. anticoagulant: general type
8. _____ abciximab (ReoPro)	b. antiplatelet type drug
9. _____ aspirin (ASA)	c. low-molecular-weight heparin (LMWH)
10. _____ enoxaparin (Lovenox)	d. ADP receptor blocker
11. _____ reteplase (Retavase)	e. glycoprotein IIb/IIIa blocker
12. _____ tirofiban (Aggrastat)	f. thrombolytic
13. _____ aminocaproic acid (Amicar)	g. hemostatic
14. _____ clopidogrel (Plavix)	

MULTIPLE CHOICE

15. Which of the following clump and adhere to the wall of an injured blood vessel to begin the process of hemostasis?

    a. Platelets

    b. Red blood cells

    c. White blood cells

    d. Antibodies

16. What is the solid, insoluble part of a blood clot called?

    a. Fibrin

    b. Thrombin

    c. Prothrombin

    d. Plasmin

17. Normal blood clotting occurs in about how many minutes?

    a. 2

    b. 3

    c. 6

    d. 10

18. Which organ is responsible for making many of the factors necessary for blood clotting?

    a. Kidney

    b. Liver

    c. Brain

    d. Skin

19. What is the process of clot removal called?

    a. Embolysis

    b. Thrombolysis

    c. Plasminolysis

    d. Fibrinolysis

20. What class of drugs promotes the formation of blood clots?

    a. Hemostatics

    b. Thrombolytics

    c. Fibrinolytics

    d. Plasminogen activators

21. The nurse is administering heparin. Which lab test should the nurse use to monitor pharmacotherapy with heparin?

    a. Bleeding time

    b. PT

    c. INR

    d. aPTT

22. Anticoagulants are drugs that do which of the following?

    a. Dissolve thrombi that have recently formed

    b. Shorten PT time

    c. Prevent thrombi from forming or growing larger

    d. Cause platelets to become less sticky

23. What is the primary advantage of using low-molecular-weight heparins (LMWHs) rather than heparin?

    a. LMWHs possess greater anticoagulant activity.

    b. LMWHs may be given by the oral route.

    c. LMWHs produce a more stable effect on coagulation; therefore, fewer lab tests are needed.

    d. LMWHs have a prolonged duration of action.

24. The nurse must monitor for which of the following serious adverse effects of anticoagulant therapy?

    a. Hemorrhage

    b. Migraines

    c. Electrolyte depletion

    d. Dysrhythmias

25. The nurse should administer which of the following antagonists, if serious hemorrhage occurs during heparin therapy?

    a. Protamine sulfate

    b. Vitamin K

    c. Adenosine diphosphate (ADP)

    d. Desmopressin (DDAVP)

26. When teaching a patient about using warfarin, the nurse should tell the patient that the anticoagulant activity can take how long to reach its maximum effect?

    a. Several minutes

    b. Several hours

    c. Several days

    d. Several weeks

27. The nurse must ensure that vitamin K is available as an antidote to treat an overdose with which of the following?

    a. Aspirin

    b. Heparin and LMWHs

    c. Aminocaproic acid (Amicar)

    d. Warfarin (Coumadin)

28. A patient has called the nurse and said that he has stopped taking warfarin because his prescription expired. The nurse should know that the pharmacologic activity of warfarin will take how long to diminish?

    a. 10 minutes

    b. 10 hours

    c. 24 hours

    d. 3 days

29. Aspirin causes its anticoagulant effect by inhibiting which of the following?

    a. Plasminogen

    b. Prothrombin

    c. Thromboxane$_2$

    d. Glycoprotein IIb/IIIa

30. Glycoprotein IIb/IIIa inhibitors act by blocking the final step in which of the following?

    a. Hemostasis

    b. Platelet aggregation

    c. Activation of plasminogen

    d. Formation of vitamin K

31. The primary action of streptokinase is to convert plasminogen to which of the following?

    a. Plasminogen activator

    b. Plasmin

    c. Fibrin

    d. Fibrinogen

32. The nurse understands that the primary action of hemostatics is to do which of the following?

    a. Dissolve thrombi

    b. Prevent thrombi

    c. Reverse the effects of anticoagulants

    d. Prevent excessive bleeding following surgery

33. Which of the following is NOT an indication for thrombolytic therapy?

    a. Acute myocardial infarction (MI)

    b. Postoperative bleeding

    c. Pulmonary embolism

    d. Deep vein thrombosis (DVT)

MAKING CONNECTIONS

34. A patient is receiving warfarin, which is 98% bound to plasma proteins. The antidepressant paroxetine (Paxil), which is 95% bound, is added to the patient's daily medications. If the paroxetine displaces warfarin from its binding sites, which of the following will most likely occur?

    a. Toxicity to warfarin

    b. Toxicity to paroxetine

    c. Diminished effect from warfarin

    d. Diminished effect from paroxetine

35. The antidepressant imipramine (Tofranil) is metabolized to its active form, desipramine, in the liver. The nurse knows that the dose of imipramine for patients with liver cirrhosis should be which of the following?

    a. Increased above average

    b. Decreased below average

    c. An average dose

    d. This patient should not receive imipramine

36. Which of the following is a widely used class of antipsychotic medications?

    a. Phenothiazines

    b. Benzodiazepines

    c. MAO inhibitors

    d. Anticholinergics

37. What is the primary goal of the nurse for patients experiencing prn pain medications?

    a. Administer the least amount of pain medication possible.

    b. Administer analgesics only when pain becomes intolerable.

    c. Ensure that dependence does not develop.

    d. Alleviate the pain.

38. Of the following four drugs, which is NOT related to the other three?

    a. Phenytoin (Dilantin)

    b. Phenobarbital (Luminal)

    c. Sumatriptan (Imitrex)

    d. Ethosuximide (Zarontin)

CALCULATIONS

39. A patient with deep vein thrombosis has orders for heparin 2,500 units per hour. The solution strength is 50,000 units in 1,000 mL D5W. Calculate the milliliter-per-hour flow rate.

40. A patient is receiving 20,000 units of heparin in 500 mL D5W. The rate is set at 30 mL/h. How many units is the patient receiving per hour? How many units will the patient receive in a day?

CASE STUDY APPLICATIONS

41. A female patient is being discharged from the hospital following surgery for replacement of a heart valve. She will be placed on long-term warfarin (Coumadin) therapy. The nurse is developing this patient's discharge teaching plan.

    a. List the activities that the nurse should teach the patient to avoid.

    b. Describe the signs and symptoms that would alert the patient to adverse effects of warfarin therapy.

    c. What medications and what herbal supplements should be avoided while the patient is being treated with warfarin?

42. A 50-year-old man is being admitted to the hospital for the third time this year. He has a history of alcohol abuse, diabetes, and heart failure. He was brought to the hospital with a complaint of abdominal pain and vomiting of bright red blood. His diagnosis is perforated gastric ulcer. The patient states that he has been taking warfarin for an irregular heartbeat and Glucophage for diabetes.

    a. With this limited admission history, what factors might have contributed to this patient's acute bleeding episode?

    b. What nursing diagnoses and patient outcomes would be essential in this situation?

    c. What medications might be ordered for this patient?

CHAPTER 31

DRUGS FOR HEMATOPOIETIC DISORDERS

FILL IN THE BLANK

From the textbook, find the correct word(s) to complete the statement(s).

1. Red blood cell formation, also known as _____, is regulated by the hormone _____.

2. Human erythropoietin is marketed as the drug _____ _____.

3. Administering oprelvekin (Neumega) will increase the number of _____ in the blood.

4. Colony stimulating factors (CSFs) are substances that regulate the number of _____ in the blood.

5. _____ and _____ maintain iron stores inside cells.

6. After erythrocytes die, most of the iron in their hemoglobin is _____ for later use.

Adams/Holland, *Student Workbook and Resource Guide for Pharmacology for Nurses* 4th Edition
© 2014 by Pearson Education, Inc.

MATCHING

For questions 7 through 14, match the indication in column I with its drug in column II.

Column I	Column II
7. _____ pernicious anemia	a. epoetin alfa (Epogen)
8. _____ anemia with HIV infection	b. filgrastim (Neupogen)
9. _____ AIDS-related immunosuppression	c. cyanocobalamin
10. _____ anemia caused by chemotherapy	d. ferrous sulfate
11. _____ neutropenia caused by chemotherapy	
12. _____ chronic renal failure	
13. _____ megaloblastic anemia	

MULTIPLE CHOICE

14. Which of the following is the most common adverse effect observed with ferrous sulfate pharmacotherapy?

    a. Decreased leukocyte counts

    b. Liver damage

    c. Retention of fluids/edema

    d. Nausea and vomiting

15. Nursing interventions for patients receiving hematopoietic growth factor therapy include all of the following EXCEPT:

    a. assessing for a history of uncontrolled hypertension.

    b. assessing for food or drug allergies.

    c. assessing for signs of liver impairment.

    d. monitoring for early signs of stroke or myocardial infarction (MI).

16. Therapeutic actions of colony-stimulating factors include all of the following EXCEPT:

    a. increased migration of leukocytes to antigens.

    b. increased effectiveness of antibodies.

    c. rapid platelet production.

    d. increased phagocytosis.

17. Patients who are neutropenic secondary to antineoplastic chemotherapy can be expected to receive which of the following?

    a. Erythropoietin

    b. Filgrastim (Neupogen)

    c. Oprelvekin (Neumega)

    d. Sargramostim (Leukine)

18. The patient is receiving an IV infusion of sargramostim (Leukine). He develops dyspnea, rapid pulse, hypotension, and complains of feeling dizzy. What should the nurse do?

    a. Call the doctor and prepare to administer epinephrine.

    b. Assess the patient for an allergy to yeast.

    c. Obtain a complete blood count (CBC) and differential.

    d. Discontinue the IV line, then restart it at half the previous rate after the symptoms are gone.

19. Patient teaching for filgrastim (Neupogen) includes all of the following EXCEPT:

    a. take medication with a full glass of water to decrease the risk of kidney damage.

    b. wash hands frequently and avoid people with infections.

    c. report chest pain, palpitations, respiratory problems, fever, chills, and malaise to the health care provider immediately.

    d. keep all laboratory and doctor appointments.

20. What is the recommended route for administering oprelvekin (Neumega)?

    a. PO

    b. IV

    c. SC

    d. IM

21. For patients receiving antineoplastic therapy, figrastim (Neupogen) should not be administered until:

    a. 24 hours after the chemotherapy session.

    b. erythrocyte counts have returned to normal levels.

    c. leukocyte counts have returned to normal levels.

    d. nausea from the chemotherapy has passed.

22. Which of the following statements about pernicious anemia is false?

    a. It affects more than one body system.

    b. The stem cells produce abnormally large leukocytes that do not fully mature.

    c. Permanent nervous system damage may result if the disease remains untreated.

    d. Intrinsic factor is required to prevent the disease.

23. Which of the following is NOT a common cause of iron deficiency?

    a. Blood loss

    b. Pregnancy

    c. Intensive athletic training

    d. Kidney disease

24. Which of these statements regarding iron preparations is false?

    a. Prior to administering an IV dose, the patient must receive a test dose.

    b. Iron should be taken with food to increase absorption.

    c. Iron may cause nausea, vomiting, and constipation.

    d. Iron may turn stools dark green or black.

25. Which of the following drugs must be given using the Z-track method?

    a. Iron dextran (Dexferrum)

    b. Cyanocobalamin

    c. Filgrastim (Neupogen)

    d. Epoetin alfa (Epogen)

26. Which of the following statements regarding folic acid is false?

    a. It does not require intrinsic factor for intestinal absorption.

    b. The most common cause of deficiency is insufficient dietary intake.

    c. Deficiency is commonly seen in chronic alcoholics.

    d. It is unsafe to take this preparation during pregnancy.

MAKING CONNECTIONS

27. An anticholinergic drug is one that blocks the effects of which of the following?

    a. Epinephrine

    b. Norepinephrine

    c. Acetylcholine

    d. Serotonin

28. Which major depolarizing neuromuscular blocker is used during surgery?

    a. Succinylcholine (Anectine)

    b. Acetylcholine

    c. Promethazine (Phenergan)

    d. Bethanechol (Urecholine)

29. Which of the following would be used to treat mild to moderate pain due to inflammation?

    a. Oxycodone (OxyContin)

    b. Meperidine (Demerol)

    c. Ibuprofen (Advil)

    d. Acetaminophen (Tylenol)

30. What antagonist may be administered if serious hemorrhage occurs during heparin therapy?

    a. Protamine sulfate

    b. Vitamin K

    c. Adenosine diphosphate (ADP)

    d. Aminocaproic acid (Amicar)

31. The nurse uses which of the following during a hypertensive emergency to lower extremely high blood pressure within minutes?

    a. Hydralazine (Apresoline)

    b. Nitroprusside (Nitropress)

    c. Doxazosin (Cardura)

    d. Prazosin (Minipress)

CALCULATIONS

32. How much filgrastim (Neupogen) would the nurse give a patient who weighs 57 kg, for whom the minimum dose of 5 mcg/kg/day is ordered subcutaneously?

33. A pediatric patient weighs 66 lb. The physician has ordered a subcutaneous daily dose of filgrastim 750 mcg. The maximum recommended subcutaneous dose is 20 mcg/kg/day. Is this dose within the recommended limits?

CASE STUDY APPLICATIONS

34. A 58-year-old male comes to the dialysis clinic three times a week. He receives Epogen injections after each treatment.

    a. What teaching can the nurse provide this patient regarding why he needs to receive erythropoietin?

    b. What adverse effects of erythropoietin should be assessed during each clinic visit?

    c. One of the nurse's goals for this patient is "to promote patient independence regarding self-care." What patient education is necessary for him?

35. A 63-year-old male has been admitted with a diagnosis of megaloblastic anemia. He complains of feeling tired and weak. He states, "I just can't make myself do anything." The patient has a history of gout and chronic gastritis. He wants to know why he is not on an iron preparation, since that is how a friend's anemia was treated. Further assessment reveals that the patient has virtually no knowledge of his disease or treatment. The nursing care plan includes teaching interventions to address this knowledge deficit.

    a. The nurse is evaluating the patient's understanding of why he feels tired and weak. What should he tell the nurse?

    b. What teaching would the nurse provide the patient regarding self-care?

    c. How would the nurse explain to the patient that an iron preparation is probably not the answer to his problem?

36. A female has been receiving chemotherapy for her cancer. She is admitted with a diagnosis of neutropenia. She has been started on filgrastim (Neupogen) injections and placed on neutropenic precautions.

    a. What assessments must the nurse make prior to giving the patient her first injection of filgrastim?

    b. What teaching would the nurse provide this patient regarding the adverse effects of her medication?

    c. While evaluating the patient's understanding of the teaching, the nurse asks the patient how she can decrease her risk of getting an infection. What should the patient be able to tell the nurse?

CHAPTER 32

DRUGS FOR IMMUNE SYSTEM MODULATION

FILL IN THE BLANK

From the textbook, find the correct word(s) to complete the statement(s).

1. B cells initiate _____ immunity and secrete _____ that neutralize or mark the antigen for destruction by other cells in the immune system.

2. When the patient's immune system is stimulated to produce antibodies due to exposure to a specific antigen, it is referred to as _____ immunity.

3. The administration of gamma globulin after exposure to hepatitis is referred to as _____ immunity.

4. Activated T cells recognize specific antigens and produce hormone-like proteins called _____ that regulate the intensity and duration of the immune response.

5. Immunostimulants, also called _____ _____ _____, have been approved to boost certain functions of the immune system.

6. Immunosuppressants are effective at inhibiting a patient's immune system, but must be monitored carefully as loss of immune function can lead to _____.

7. Four drug classes used to dampen the immune response are _____, _____, _____, and _____ _____.

Adams/Holland, *Student Workbook and Resource Guide for Pharmacology for Nurses* 4th Edition
© 2014 by Pearson Education, Inc.

MATCHING

For questions 8 through 13, match the drug in column I to the primary class in column II.

Column I	Column II
8. _____ interferon alfa-2b (Intron A)	a. calcineurin inhibitor
9. _____ cyclosporine (Neoral, Sandimmune)	b. immune globulin preparation
10. _____ human papillomavirus (Cervarix, Gardasil)	c. immunostimulant
11. _____ basiliximab (Simulect)	d. vaccine
12. _____ azathioprine (Imuran)	e. antibody
13. _____ cytomegalovirus immune globulin (CytoGam)	f. antimetabolite/cytotoxic agent

MULTIPLE CHOICE

14. Foreign substances or cells that elicit a specific immune response are referred to as which of the following?

    a. Immunoglobulins

    b. Cytokines

    c. Antigens

    d. Antibodies

15. A nurse must understand the interrelationships in the immune system. One of those relationships is that the primary function of plasma cells is to secrete which of the following?

    a. Complement

    b. Histamine

    c. Antibodies

    d. Cytokines

16. Memory B cells are programmed to remember the initial antigen interaction. Should the body be exposed to the same antigen in the future, the body manufactures high levels of antibodies in approximately what time frame?

    a. 2 to 3 hours

    b. 2 to 3 days

    c. 2 to 3 weeks

    d. 2 to 3 months

17. Which class of drugs is administered to prevent the body's rejection of an organ transplant?

    a. COX-2 inhibitors

    b. H_2-receptor antagonists

    c. Immunosuppressants

    d. Interferons

18. Which drug produces its therapeutic effects by inhibiting T cells?

    a. Cyclosporine (Sandimmune)

    b. Prednisone

    c. Aspirin

    d. Celecoxib (Celebrex)

19. The nurse is administering the patient 18 mg/kg of cyclosporine. The nurse should monitor the patient for primary adverse effects relating to which system?

    a. Immune system

    b. Lung

    c. GI tract

    d. Kidney

20. Which is NOT a type of vaccine suspension?

    a. Live microbes

    b. Killed microbes

    c. Microbes that are alive but attenuated

    d. Bacterial toxins

21. To present effective patient education, the nurse must know that the purpose of a vaccine is which of the following?

    a. To treat active infections

    b. To prevent inflammation, should an infection occur

    c. To prevent infections from occurring

    d. To suppress the immune system so that hypersensitivity to antigens does not occur

22. When providing patient education, the nurse needs to understand that a toxoid is classified as which of the following?

    a. Vaccine

    b. Immunosuppressant

    c. Anti-inflammatory agent

    d. Antigen

23. Which biologic response modifier would be prescribed for the treatment of Kaposi's sarcoma?

    a. Interleukin-2

    b. Interleukin-11

    c. Interferon alfa-2b

    d. Interferon beta

24. Which biologic response modifier would be prescribed for the treatment of metastatic renal carcinoma?

    a. Interleukin-2

    b. Interleukin-11

   c. Interferon alfa-2b

   d. Interferon beta

25. Which biologic response modifier is reserved for the treatment of severe multiple sclerosis?

   a. Interleukin-2

   b. Interleukin-11

   c. Interferon alfa-2b

   d. Interferon beta

MAKING CONNECTIONS

26. Which drug administration method has the highest potential for severe adverse effects?

   a. PO

   b. IM

   c. IV

   d. SC

27. Lisinopril (Prinivil) and quinapril (Accupril) belong to a class of drugs called:

   a. calcium channel blockers

   b. beta adrenergic blockers

   c. ACE inhibitors

   d. alpha adrenergic blockers

28. A patient receiving atomoxetine (Strattera) is most likely being treated for which disorder?

   a. Clinical depression

   b. Bipolar disorder

   c. Psychosis

   d. Attention deficit/hyperactivity disorder

29. Which is a potential early adverse effect from nitrous oxide?

   a. Restlessness or anxiety

   b. Dysrhythmia

   c. Hypertension

   d. Mania

30. Which primary action of digoxin (Lanoxin) is effective in the treatment of heart failure?

   a. It dilates the coronary arteries.

   b. It increases cardiac conduction.

   c. It decreases blood pressure.

   d. It increases cardiac contractility/output.

CALCULATIONS

31. A patient is to receive cytomegalovirus immune globulin (CytoGam). The order reads: to be given IV 150 mg/kg within 72 hours of transplantation, then 100 mg/kg 2, 4, 6, and 8 wk post-transplant, then 50 mg/kg 12 and 16 wk post transplant. The patient weighs 180 lb. How many milligrams will he receive in 72 hours, 2, 4, 6, 8, 12, and 16 wk?

32. A female patient is to receive tacrolimus (Prograf) 0.15 mg/kg/day every 12 h. She weighs 100 lb. How many milligrams will she receive in 12 hours and in 24 hours?

CASE STUDY APPLICATIONS

33. A female patient has been diagnosed with hairy cell leukemia, and it has been recommended that she begin receiving immunostimulant therapy. During the initial physical assessment, it was determined that she is 6 weeks pregnant. Because the physician has determined that interferon beta-1b is the appropriate drug for this condition, the nurse must carefully monitor the patient for signs of complications related to the drug therapy and status of the pregnancy.

    a. What possible adverse reaction can this drug have on pregnancy?

    b. What complications and/or adverse reactions do immunostimulants cause?

    c. What side effects should patients taking immunostimulants be instructed to report to their primary nurse?

34. A female patient recently received a kidney transplant and is being released to go home. The nurse discharging her determines that extensive patient education regarding the purpose, action, and possible adverse reactions to immunosuppressants is necessary for the future well-being of this patient.

    a. What is the purpose of immunosuppressants, and for how long will it be necessary for the patient to receive this drug therapy?

    b. Explain the action of this class of drugs.

    c. What are the possible adverse reactions to this drug therapy?

35. A 1-year-old boy has just received his measles, mumps, and rubella (MMR II) vaccine. His mother is not sure why her son needs to have "all of these shots." The nurse explains to the child's mother the rationale for her son receiving the vaccinations. The nurse also presents information on the possible adverse reactions and explains that severe reactions to vaccinations are rare.

    a. What rationale would the nurse give the mother for the vaccinations?

    b. For what adverse reactions would the nurse teach the mother to monitor?

CHAPTER 33

DRUGS FOR INFLAMMATION AND FEVER

FILL IN THE BLANK

From the textbook, find the correct word(s) to complete the statement(s).

1. The primary purpose of inflammation is to _____.

2. _____ cells detect foreign agents or injury and respond by releasing histamine.

3. Tinnitus, dizziness, headache, and excessive sweating are signs of a condition called _____.

4. The primary drug class used for the treatment of mild to moderate inflammation is the _____ _____ _____ _____.

5. _____ are natural hormones released by the adrenal cortex that have powerful effects on nearly every cell in the body.

6. During long-term therapy with corticosteroids the nurse must be alert for signs of a condition called _____ syndrome.

7. Aspirin is avoided in pediatric patients younger than age 18 who present with fever because of the possibility of _____ syndrome.

Adams/Holland, *Student Workbook and Resource Guide for Pharmacology for Nurses* 4th Edition
© 2014 by Pearson Education, Inc.

MATCHING

For questions 8 through 14, match the primary class in column I with its drug in column II.

Column I	Column II
8. _____ dexamethasone	a. ibuprofen-like drug
9. _____ fenoprofen (Nalfon)	b. selective COX-2 inhibitor
10. _____ oxaprozin (Daypro)	c. corticosteroid
11. _____ prednisolone	d. salicylate
12. _____ celecoxib (Celebrex)	
13. _____ aspirin	
14. _____ triamcinolone (Kenalog)	

MULTIPLE CHOICE

15. The nurse would determine that the use of hydrocortisone would be contraindicated in a patient experiencing which of the following?

    a. An active infection associated with inflammation

    b. Pain associated with inflammation

    c. Nasal congestion

    d. Hypertension

16. What is the primary action of histamine?

    a. Vasodilator

    b. Vasoconstrictor

    c. Sympathomimetic

    d. Cardiotonic agent

17. Rapid release of histamine on a massive scale throughout the body is responsible for which of the following?

    a. Irreversible inhibition of cyclooxygenase

    b. Allergic rhinitis

    c. Immunosuppression

    d. Anaphylaxis

18. Which drug does NOT exert an anti-inflammatory effect?

    a. Aspirin

    b. Ibuprofen

    c. Acetaminophen

    d. COX-2 inhibitors

19. The nurse administering high doses of aspirin should look for primary adverse effects related to which body system?

    a. GI

    b. Cardiovascular

    c. Endocrine

    d. Nervous

20. What is the primary advantage of using the selective COX-2 inhibitors over aspirin?

    a. They are less expensive.

    b. They are more effective.

    c. They have fewer adverse effects on the digestive system.

    d. They have greater anticoagulant effects.

21. If administered over a long period, which class of drugs has the potential to suppress the normal functions of the adrenal gland?

    a. NSAIDs

    b. H_2-receptor antagonists

    c. Immunosuppressants

    d. Corticosteroids

22. Which drug class is most effective at relieving severe inflammation?

    a. NSAIDs

    b. Systemic corticosteroids

    c. H_2-receptor antagonists

    d. COX-2 inhibitors

23. The patient is discharged with a prescription for naproxen 500 mg bid. The nurse should teach the patient that the most common adverse effect of this drug is:

    a. rash.

    b. nausea/vomiting.

    c. headache.

    d. possible infections.

24. Corticosteroids have many indications. Which of the following is NOT an indication for drugs in this class?

    a. Neoplasia

    b. Arthritis

    c. Asthma

    d. Pain

MAKING CONNECTIONS

25. A nurse notes in the patient's chart that he is receiving risperidone. This patient is most likely being treated for which condition?

    a. insomnia

    b. schizophrenia

    c. bipolar disorder

    d. fibromyalgia

26. For which condition is phenytoin (Dilantin) most frequently used?

    a. Bipolar disorder

    b. Migraines

    c. Schizophrenia

    d. Seizures

27. Which organ is responsible for the first-pass effect?

    a. Liver

    b. Brain

    c. Kidneys

    d. Small intestine

28. Which of the following is an opioid?

    a. Hydralazine

    b. Hydrocortisone

    c. Hydrocodone

    d. Hydrochlorothiazide

29. Which of the following is the most common adverse effect of cholestyramine?

    a. Hypotension

    b. Drowsiness

    c. Bloating, nausea, or constipation

    d. Increased LDL levels

CALCULATIONS

30. A mother is to give her son Tylenol 30 gtt PO every 4 hours for elevated temperature. How many milliliters would she give her son in one dose? What would be the total gtt and milliliters given in 24 hours?

31. A physician has prescribed naproxen for stiff and painful joints. The order reads "Naprosyn 500 mg PO qid." The pharmacy sends 250-mg tablets. How many tablet(s) would the patient receive in one dose? How many milligrams will he receive in a 24-hour period, and would the amount be within the recommended dosage for a 24-hour period?

CASE STUDY APPLICATIONS

32. An 18-year-old man presents to the emergency department (ED) on a Sunday complaining of a severe toothache. During examination, the nurse notes an abscess surrounding a molar that is red, swollen, and inflamed. The patient also presents with a temperature of 39°C. Based on the presenting symptoms, the ARNP suspects a systemic bacterial infection and prescribes the following medications:

   Ampicillin

   Empirin 2

   Ketoprofen (Orudis)

   The in-house pharmacy fills the prescriptions, but assigns the patient education related to drug therapy to the nurse in charge of the outpatient.

   a. Explain the therapeutic rationale for Empirin 2 and ketoprofen.

   b. Explain why the ARNP did not prescribe a corticosteroid to reduce the inflammation.

   c. Explain the most common adverse reactions to Empirin 2 and ketoprofen.

33. A 64-year-old woman presents with the complaint of stiff and painful joints in both hands. The health care provider has prescribed Celebrex. The patient education for this condition should include potential adverse reactions to the class of medications and when to notify the provider in relationship to these adverse reactions. The patient should also receive information on nonpharmacologic methods to reduce symptoms of the condition.

   a. Determine the drug classification.

   b. Why are the medications in this drug class the preferred drugs for the treatment of inflammation?

   c. What should the nurse assess prior to the patient receiving any drug from this classification?

34. A mother has brought her 6-month-old son into the ED with a temperature of 103.7°F. The health care provider orders Tylenol infant drops to reduce the temperature. The mother is 17 years old, and a first-time mother, without a support system at home. She looks to the nurse for information on the proper method to administer the medication to her son.

   a. Why did the provider order Tylenol and not aspirin?

   b. Why did the provider order infant drops?

   c. What disorder can be acquired in young children receiving aspirin therapy?

CHAPTER 34

DRUGS FOR BACTERIAL INFECTIONS

FILL IN THE BLANK

From the textbook, find the correct word(s) to complete the statement(s).

1. A highly _____ microbe is one that can produce disease when present in very small numbers.

2. Genetic errors referred to as _____ commonly occur in bacterial cells and may result in drug resistance.

3. When anti-infectives are effective against a wide variety of microorganisms, they are classified as _____ _____.

4. A _____ is a type of infection that occurs secondary to anti-infective drug therapy.

5. _____ is an enzyme secreted by bacteria that limits the therapeutic usefulness of penicillins.

6. Augmentin, Timentin, and Unasyn are combination drugs that contain a penicillin and a _____ _____.

7. _____ antibiotics are safe alternatives to penicillin because they can generally be administered over a shorter time.

8. Narrow-spectrum antibiotics classified as _____ are useful for the treatment of serious gram-negative infections, but they also have the potential for producing ear and kidney toxicity.

Adams/Holland, *Student Workbook and Resource Guide for Pharmacology for Nurses* 4th Edition
© 2014 by Pearson Education, Inc.

MATCHING

For questions 9 through 18, match the type of medication in column I with its pharmacologic category in column II.

Column I	Column II
9. _____ amoxicillin (Amoxil, Trimox)	a. penicillin
10. _____ ciprofloxacin (Cipro)	b. cephalosporin
11. _____ cefepime (Maxipime)	c. tetracycline
12. _____ gentamicin (Garamycin)	d. macrolide
13. _____ neomycin	e. aminoglycoside
14. _____ erythromycin (E-Mycin)	f. fluoroquinolone or miscellaneous
15. _____ doxycycline (Vibramycin)	g. antitubercular agent
16. _____ cephalexin (Keflex)	
17. _____ rifampin (Rifadin, Rimactane)	
18. _____ vancomycin (Vancocin)	

For questions 19 through 25, match the organism in column I with its disease(s) in column II.

Column I	Column II
19. _____ *Neisseria*	a. venereal disease, endometriosis
20. _____ *Pseudomonas*	b. urinary tract infection (UTI), skin infections
21. _____ *Rickettsia*	c. traveler's diarrhea, UTI, bacteremia, endometriosis
22. _____ *Klebsiella*	d. pharyngitis, pneumonia, skin infections, septicemia, endocarditis
23. _____ *Borrelia*	e. Lyme disease
24. _____ *Escherichia*	f. Rocky Mountain spotted fever
25. _____ *Chlamydia*	

MULTIPLE CHOICE

26. What is the advantage of using an antibiotic that is classified as a broad-spectrum antibiotic?

    a. It produces fewer adverse effects.

    b. It is effective against a small number of organisms.

    c. It is effective against a large number of organisms.

    d. It has a greater potency.

27. What is the action of bacteriocidal drugs?

    a. They have a high potency.

    b. They have high efficacy.

c. They kill the infectious agent.

d. They slow the growth of the infectious agent.

28. What is the advantage of using amoxicillin (Amoxil, Trimox) over penicillin G?

    a. Less expensive

    b. Greater absorption

    c. Fewer adverse effects

    d. Penicillinase resistance

29. Which class of antibiotics is usually reserved for urinary tract infections and has serious adverse effects on hearing and kidney function?

    a. Erythromycin

    b. Aminoglycoside

    c. Tetracycline

    d. Sulfonamide

30. Which antibiotic is known as the "last chance" drug, for treatment of resistant infections?

    a. Clarithromycin (Biaxin)

    b. Dicloxacillin

    c. Vancomycin (Vancocin)

    d. Trimethoprim-sulfamethoxazole (Bactrim, Septra)

31. Which antibiotic would most likely be used for a patient who is to receive dental surgery who is allergic to penicillin?

    a. Clindamycin (Cleocin)

    b. Amoxicillin (Amoxil, Trimox)

    c. Sulfisoxazole (Gantrisin)

    d. Erythromycin (E-Mycin)

32. Which drug class acts by inhibiting the metabolism of folic acid by bacteria?

    a. Aminoglycosides

    b. Tetracyclines

    c. Sulfonamides

    d. Macrolides

33. Photosensitivity and teeth discoloration are potential adverse effects with which of the following?

    a. Aminoglycosides

    b. Metronidazole (Flagyl)

    c. Cephalosporins

    d. Tetracyclines

34. Which of the following is a preferred drug for the treatment of *M. tuberculosis*?

    a. Erythromycin (E-Mycin, Erythrocin)

    b. Gentamicin (Garamycin)

    c. Vancomycin (Vancocin)

    d. Isoniazid (INH)

35. Which of the following is an antibiotic responsible for causing red-man syndrome as an adverse effect?

    a. Cefotaxime (Claforan)

    b. Tetracycline

    c. Erythromycin (E-Mycin, Erythrocin)

    d. Vancomycin (Vancocin)

36. How does drug therapy of tuberculosis differ from that of most other infections?

    a. Patients with tuberculosis have no symptoms.

    b. Mycobacteria have a cell wall that is resistant to penetration by anti-infective drugs.

    c. Patients usually require therapy for a shorter time.

    d. Antituberculosis drugs are used extensively for treating the disease, not preventing it.

37. What is the purpose of culture and sensitivity testing?

    a. To prevent an infection, a practice called chemoprophylaxis

    b. To determine which antibiotic is most effective against the infecting microorganism

    c. To prevent acquired resistance

    d. To promote the development of drug-resistant bacterial strains by killing the bacteria sensitive to a drug

38. Which of the following types of antibiotics are more likely to cause superinfections?

    a. Narrow-spectrum antibiotics

    b. Broad-spectrum antibiotics

    c. Original penicillin

    d. Bacteriostatic drugs

39. Which antibiotic class is one of the oldest, safest and effective, although widespread resistance has developed to the drugs?

    a. Penicillins

    b. Tetracyclines

    c. Macrolides

    d. Aminoglycosides

40. All of the following are first-line drugs for treating tuberculosis EXCEPT:

    a. pyrazinamide (PZA)

    b. rifabutin (Mycobutin)

    c. ethambutol (Myambutol)

    d. metronidazole (Flagyl)

MAKING CONNECTIONS

41. Which local anesthetic drug might interfere with the antibacterial activity of some sulfonamide drugs?

    a. Benzocaine (Americaine)

    b. Tetracaine (Pontocaine)

    c. Bupivacaine (Marcaine)

    d. Lidocaine (Xylocaine)

42. Which action might influence antibiotic absorption within the stomach?

    a. Taking an antacid along with the antibiotic

    b. Drinking a glass of water with the antibiotic

    c. Taking an antibiotic suspension without shaking up the medicine vial

    d. Taking the antibiotic just before going to bed

43. If convulsive seizures were to develop with antibiotic therapy, which symptoms would most likely NOT be observed?

    a. Jerking muscular movements

    b. Difficulty breathing and biting the tongue

    c. Blank stare with psychotic symptoms

    d. Loss of bladder control

44. Following oral administration, chlorpromazine (Thorazine) is rapidly inactivated by the liver. What is this inactivation called?

    a. Enterohepatic recirculation

    b. First-pass effect

    c. Gastric–hepatic barrier

    d. Enzyme induction

45. Which term is NOT associated with the drug levodopa (Dopar)?

    a. Anticholinergic

    b. Anti-Parkinson's agent

    c. Dopamine

    d. Sympathomimetic

CALCULATIONS

46. A patient is to receive amoxicillin 500 mg PO every 6 hours for 7 days. The pharmacy sends to the floor amoxicillin 1 g in scored tablets. How many tablet(s) will the patient receive in each dose? How many tablet(s) will the patient receive in a 12-hour period?

47. A patient is receiving ciprofloxacin (Cipro) for a urinary tract infection (UTI). The order reads: Cipro 500 mg PO qid for 5 days. The pharmacy sends Cipro 250 mg. How many tablet(s) will the patient receive in a 24-hour period?

CASE STUDY APPLICATIONS

48. For several years, a female patient has taken antibiotics on a frequent basis for kidney infections. She has been informed by the nurse that she is likely to develop a drug-resistant infection.

    a. What are the potential results of the widespread use of antibiotics?

    b. What is the relationship between the long-term use of antibiotics and resistant strains of bacteria?

    c. What is the potential problem that the patient may develop?

    d. What will happen to the therapeutic effect of the antibiotic?

49. A male patient has been diagnosed with bacterial pneumonia and has been treated with a broad-spectrum antibiotic until the bacteria can be isolated and the appropriate drug administered. The patient asks the nurse the rationale for starting him on one antibiotic when the drug therapy may be changed after lab results have isolated the bacteria.

    a. Why are broad-spectrum antibiotics sometimes prescribed?

    b. What tests must be done to identify the microbe?

    c. What changes in treatment will be recommended after the microbe is identified?

50. An 88-year-old patient with impaired renal function has been diagnosed with a urinary tract infection (UTI). The patient has been receiving a sulfonamide, but his primary health care provider has determined that this is not an appropriate course of treatment for him. Examine the factors that support this decision and the potential adverse effects that might be expected if the treatment continues.

    a. What are the potential adverse effects of sulfonamides?

    b. What is the nurse's role in sulfonamide therapy?

    c. How does sulfonamide therapy affect the patient's intake of fluids?

CHAPTER 35

DRUGS FOR FUNGAL, PROTOZOAN, AND HELMINTHIC INFECTIONS

FILL IN THE BLANK

From the textbook, find the correct word(s) to complete the statement(s).

1. _____ are single-celled or multicellular organisms that are more complex than bacteria.

2. Patients with healthy immune defenses are afflicted with community-acquired infections such as _____, _____, _____, and _____.

3. Opportunistic fungal infections acquired in a nosocomial setting will more likely be _____, _____, _____, and _____.

4. Fungal infections are called _____.

5. Superficial fungal infections are sometimes referred to as _____.

6. Systemic fungal infections typically affect organs such as the _____, _____, and _____ _____.

7. Some of the newer antifungal agents may be used for either _____ or _____ infections.

8. The largest class of antifungals, the _____, inhibits _____ which is an essential component of fungal cell membranes, synthesis, causing the fungal plasma membrane to become porous or leaky.

9. _____ is the traditional drug for the treatment of serious systemic fungal infections.

10. The major advantage of the azoles is that they may be administered _____.

Adams/Holland, *Student Workbook and Resource Guide for Pharmacology for Nurses* 4th Edition
© 2014 by Pearson Education, Inc.

MATCHING

For questions 11 through 16, match the name of the fungus in column I with whether it usually causes a systemic or topical infection in column II.

Column I	Column II
11. _____ *Aspergillus fumigatus*	a. systemic infection
12. _____ *Epidermophyton floccosum*	b. topical infection
13. _____ *Coccidioides immitis*	
14. _____ *Histoplasma capsulatum*	
15. _____ *Sporothrix schenckii*	
16. _____ *Pneumocystis jiroveci*	

For questions 17 through 22, match the antifungal drug in column I with its indication in column II.

Column I	Column II
17. _____ butoconazole (Femstat)	a. skin mycoses
18. _____ econazole (Spectazole)	b. ringworm, skin, and nail infections
19. _____ flucytosine (Ancobon)	c. vaginal mycoses
20. _____ griseofulvin (Fulvicin)	d. severe systemic infections
21. _____ nystatin (Mycostatin, others)	e. candidiasis
22. _____ undecylenic acid (Fungi-Nail)	f. athlete's foot, diaper rash

MULTIPLE CHOICE

23. Systemic mycoses are frequently quite severe and affect more than one body system. These mycoses often require which treatment(s)?

    a. Topical agents only

    b. Oral medications only

    c. Parenteral medications only

    d. Oral and parenteral medications

24. The nurse is administering fluconazole (Diflucan) PO for vaginal candidiasis. The nurse should teach the patient that the most frequent side effect of this drug is:

    a. superinfection of the vagina

    b. headaches

    c. liver toxicity

    d. nausea/vomiting and diarrhea

25. Which drug is NOT indicated for systemic fungal infections?

    a. Fluconazole (Diflucan)

    b. Caspofungin (Cancidas)

    c. Sertaconazole (Ertaczo)

    d. Amphotericin B (Abelcet, others)

26. Candidiasis affects the skin, vagina, and mouth. Which drug is used to treat this condition and is available in a wide variety of formulations including cream, ointment, powder, tablets, and lozenges?

    a. Butenafine (Mentax)

    b. Ciclopirox (Loprox)

    c. Nystatin (Mycostatin)

    d. Terconazole (Terazol)

27. The nurse is administering an IV of amphotericin B for a severe fungal infection of the bowel. The nurse should monitor for which most common adverse effect of systemic amphotericin B therapy?

    a. Phlebitis

    b. Hypertension

    c. Gastric reflux

    d. Dryness of the mouth

28. While obtaining a history, the patient reports taking griseofulvin (Fulvicin) for 6 weeks. The nurse understands that this patient is being treated for what type of infection?

    a. Superficial fungal infection

    b. Helminthic infection

    c. Malaria

    d. Systemic fungal infection

29. Which medication would be most likely to be used in the treatment of travelers' diarrhea, a condition caused by protozoans?

    a. Doxycycline hyclate (Vibramycin)

    b. Mebendazole (Vermox)

    c. Chloroquine (Aralen)

    d. Metronidazole (Flagyl)

30. Which medication is an older, traditional drug of choice for the treatment of malaria?

    a. Praziquantel (Biltricide)

    b. Chloroquine (Aralen)

    c. Melarsoprol (Arsobal)

    d. Trimetrexate (Neutrexin)

31. Which organ(s) does amebiasis invade and cause severe ulcers and/or abscesses?

    a. Large intestine and liver

    b. Small intestine

    c. Heart

    d. Kidney and heart

32. What is the preferred drug for the treatment of most forms of amebiasis?

    a. Mebendazole (Vermox)

    b. Amphotericin (Abelcet, others)

    c. Metronidazole (Flagyl)

    d. Chloroquine (Aralen)

33. The nurse is preparing to treat a patient for a helminthic infection. What is the preferred drug for the treatment of most helminthic infections?

    a. Mebendazole (Vermox)

    b. Amphotericin (Abelcet, others)

    c. Metronidazole (Flagyl)

    d. Chloroquine (Aralen)

34. Patient education for the treatment of helminthic infections should include which of the following?

    a. Instruct the patient to stop the drug therapy as soon as he or she feels better.

    b. Instruct the patient that all family members need to be treated at the same time to prevent reinfestation.

    c. Instruct the patient to wear tight underwear.

    d. Instruct the patient not to wash bedding until drug regimen is completed.

35. What sociologic factor would the nurse need to evaluate in relationship to parasitic infections?

    a. Upper-middle-class lifestyle

    b. Good personal hygiene

    c. Poverty-level income

    d. Single-parent family

MAKING CONNECTIONS

36. The nurse should teach patients receiving thiazide diuretics for hypertension to:

    a. change positions slowly.

    b. limit consumption of potassium-rich foods.

    c. increase consumption of sodium-rich foods.

    d. discontinue taking the medication if adverse effects occur.

37. The nurse administering ferrous sulfate should monitor for the most common adverse effects of the drug that affect the:

    a. heart.

    b. gastrointestinal tract.

    c. blood.

    d. liver.

38. Calcium channel blockers are used for their effects on the:

    a. myocardium.

    b. skeletal muscle.

    c. autonomic nervous system.

    d. renal tubule.

39. A patient who is allergic to penicillin G has the potential for cross allergy to which of the following?

    a. Ampicillin

    b. Tetracycline

    c. Ciprofloxacin (Cipro)

    d. Vancomycin (Vancocin)

40. To what drug classification does ibuprofen belong?

    a. Salicylate

    b. Opioid

    c. Selective COX-2 inhibitor

    d. NSAID

CALCULATIONS

41. The physician has ordered amphotericin B, 0.25 mg/kg daily for a patient weighing 150 lb. What is the patient's weight in kilograms? How many milligrams of medication will the patient receive a day?

42. Fluconazole (Diflucan) has been ordered to treat a patient's yeast infection. The order reads 200 mg PO on day 1 to be followed by 100 mg PO daily for a total drug regimen of 2 weeks. What is the total number of milligrams the patient will receive daily after day 1?

CASE STUDY APPLICATIONS

43. A patient is 38 weeks pregnant and displays the symptoms of vaginal candidiasis. The apparent infection is not serious, but it is a concern to the nurse. Patient education regarding treatment is a priority for this patient related to the pregnancy.

    a. What approach should the patient take to have this infection treated?

    b. What precautions should be considered during the treatment?

44. A male patient has just returned from an extended trip to South America and has been diagnosed with malaria. The primary nursing consideration for this patient is education and monitoring for potential adverse reactions to the drug therapy.

    a. What is the recommended drug regimen for malaria?

    b. What are the potential adverse reactions to the recommended drug regimen?

45. A female patient has also returned from an extended vacation in Latin America and displays the symptoms of amebiasis. The nurse must understand the progression of this disease to carefully monitor this patient's condition. The nurse must also be sure that the patient receives education in relationship to the drug regimen.

    a. What drug regimen will the patient receive for this condition?

    b. What are the most common adverse reactions to this drug regimen?

    c. Amebiasis is primarily a disease of what organ?

CHAPTER 36

DRUGS FOR VIRAL INFECTIONS

FILL IN THE BLANK

From the textbook, find the correct word(s) to complete the statement(s).

1. The basic structure of a virus includes the outer protein coat or the _____, and the inner genetic materials in the form of _____ _____ or _____ _____.

2. Viruses are considered _____ _____; therefore, they require a host to replicate.

3. During the _____ stage of human immunodeficiency virus (HIV) infection, the patient is asymptomatic and may not be aware of the infection.

4. The classification of medications used to block components of the replication cycle of HIV is _____.

5. The standard aggressive treatment for HIV-AIDS using as many as four drugs concurrently is called _____ _____ _____ _____.

6. Oseltamivir (Tamiflu) and zanamivir (Relenza) are examples of a classification of drugs called the _____ _____ and are used to treat active influenza infection.

7. Lopinavir with ritonavir (Kaletra) is the prototype drug for the class of antiretrovirals called the _____ _____.

8. Hepatitis B (HBV) is caused by a _____ virus and is transmitted primarily through exposure to _____ _____ and _____ _____.

Adams/Holland, *Student Workbook and Resource Guide for Pharmacology for Nurses* 4th Edition
© 2014 by Pearson Education, Inc.

9. _____ is the drug most often prescribed for the treatment of herpesvirus infections.

10. Ribaviron (Rebetrol) is currently used for the treatment of chronic _____ infection.

MATCHING

For questions 11 through 15, match the description in column I with the term in column II.

Column I	Column II
11. _____ nucleoside reverse transcriptase inhibitors	a. HAART
12. _____ nonnucleoside reverse transcriptase inhibitors	b. capsid
13. _____ protein coat	c. NRTI
14. _____ mature infective particle	d. NNRTI
15. _____ highly active antiretroviral therapy	e. virion

MULTIPLE CHOICE

16. Which drug used to treat HIV-AIDS is a nonnucleoside reverse transcriptase inhibitor?

    a. Zidovudine (Retrovir, AZT)

    b. Nevirapine (Viramune)

    c. Lamivudine (Epivir, 3TC)

    d. Indinavir (Crixivan)

17. Acyclovir (Zovirax) is an effective treatment for all of the following EXCEPT:

    a. herpes simplex viruses (HSV) types 1 and 2.

    b. cytomegalovirus (CMV).

    c. varicella-zoster virus.

    d. Epstein–Barr virus.

18. The nurse should teach adult patients that the best approach to influenza treatment is:

    a. receive an annual vaccination.

    b. Amantadine (Symmetrel).

    c. Oseltamivir (Tamiflu).

    d. avoid large crowds.

19. The nurse is treating a patient who recently acquired an HIV infection. Which of the following is true regarding current HIV pharmacotherapy?

    a. Patients with HIV are able to live symptom-free much longer.

    b. Complete cures are now possible using highly active antiretroviral therapy (HAART).

      c. Drugs have been developed that are effective against multiple resistant HIV strains.

      d. Drugs have become available that treat the HIV-infected mother without affecting the newborn.

20. What is the purpose of HAART?

      a. To eliminate the virus from the blood

      b. To isolate HIV to the lymph nodes

      c. To reduce plasma HIV RNA to its lowest possible level

      d. All of the above

21. All of the following are classes of medications used to treat HIV-AIDS EXCEPT:

      a. nonnucleoside reverse transcriptase inhibitors (NNRTIs).

      b. nucleoside reverse transcriptase inhibitors (NRTIs).

      c. fusion inhibitors.

      d. DNA synthesis inhibitors.

22. The nurse treating a patient with zidovudine (Retrovir, AZT) should monitor for which major adverse effect?

      a. Reduced numbers of red and white blood cells

      b. Painful inflammation of blood vessels at the site of infusion

      c. Nephrotoxicity

      d. Hypertension

23. The nurse should instruct the patient receiving NRTIs to report which adverse effects?

      a. Rash, abdominal pain, nausea, vomiting, numbness, or generalized fatigue

      b. Fever, chills, blistering of the skin, reddening of the skin, muscle or joint pain

      c. Headache, insomnia, fever, constipation, frequent infections, fainting, or visual changes

      d. None of the above

24. The nurse should instruct the patient receiving NNRTIs to report which adverse effects?

      a. Rash, abdominal pain, nausea, vomiting, numbness, or generalized fatigue

      b. Fever, chills, blistering of the skin, reddening of the skin, muscle or joint pain

      c. Headache, insomnia, fever, constipation, frequent infections, fainting, or visual changes

      d. None of the above

25. The nurse should instruct the patient receiving protease inhibitors to report which adverse effects?

      a. Rash, abdominal pain, nausea, vomiting, numbness, or generalized fatigue

      b. Fever, chills, blistering of the skin, reddening of the skin, muscle or joint pain

      c. Headache, insomnia, fever, constipation, frequent infections, or visual changes

      d. None of the above

26. The nurse is treating a patient with a hepatitis C infection with peginterferon alfa-2a (Pegasys). The nurse understands that PEG (polyethylene glycol) was added to the interferon molecule to:

    a. lengthen the duration of action of the drug.

    b. reduce the development of resistant viruses during therapy.

    c. enable the drug to be given by the oral route.

    d. reduce the incidence of acute infusion-related anaphylaxis.

MAKING CONNECTIONS

27. Which drugs or class of drugs induces hepatic microsomal enzymes, resulting in drug–drug interactions?

    a. Aspirin

    b. Phenobarbital

    c. Phenothiazines

    d. Opioids

28. A drug that increases the renal reabsorption of an antiviral medication would have what affect?

    a. Increase the half-life of the antiviral

    b. Decrease the half-life of the antiviral

    c. No effect on the half-life of the antiviral

    d. Increase excretion

29. Drugs from which class can mask the signs and symptoms of a serious viral infection?

    a. Beta-adrenergic blockers

    b. Benzodiazepines

    c. Corticosteroids

    d. Phenothiazines

30. Naproxen (Naprosyn) is classified as which of the following?

    a. Salicylate

    b. Selective COX-2 inhibitor

    c. Opioid

    d. NSAID

31. The nurse would administer which drug to stimulate the production of platelets?

    a. Epoetin alfa (Epogen)

    b. Filgrastim (Neupogen)

    c. Cyanocobalamin (Cyanabin)

    d. Oprelvekin (Neumega)

CALCULATIONS

32. A female patient is to receive amantadine (Symmetrel) 100 mg PO bid 5 days for an episode of influenza. The pharmacy has only 50-mg tablets on hand. How many tablets would this patient receive per dose? How many tablets would she receive per day?

33. A male patient is to receive 9 mcg interferon alfacon-1 (Infergen) subcutaneously three times/week for 24 weeks for hepatitis B. The pharmacy has only Infergen 20 mcg/mL in stock. How many milliliters would the patient receive and what type of syringe would be used to measure the medication?

CASE STUDY APPLICATIONS

34. A male patient is HIV positive and was told that combination drug therapy would be more effective for this infection than a single drug. The nurse should teach the patient the rationale behind this type of drug therapy, the class of the drugs, and their individual actions. The nurse must remember that patient education must be explained in terms that the patient can understand.

    a. Why is combination drug therapy more effective against HIV?

    b. What are the drugs classes used in the combination therapy?

    c. What is the action of each drug?

35. A woman is in her third trimester of pregnancy with her first child, and her delivery date is late fall. Her health care provider has recommended that she take the influenza vaccination. Assess the rationale for this recommendation based on the information known at this time.

    a. What is the rationale for the patient's provider recommending the influenza vaccination?

    b. How long is the vaccination effective?

    c. Which antiviral drug has been used for many years to prevent and treat influenza?

36. A male patient has been diagnosed with hepatitis B. His health care provider has informed him that this disease causes inflammation and necrosis of the liver. The nurse in charge of patient education for this patient has determined that he should be aware of symptoms displayed with his condition and also how it can be transmitted to others.

    a. How is this disease transmitted?

    b. What are the symptoms displayed with acute hepatitis B?

    c. What are the symptoms displayed with chronic hepatitis B?

    d. What is the current recommendation for the hepatitis B vaccination?

37. A female patient has been diagnosed with genital herpes. She also is 3 months pregnant. The nurse in charge of this patient must be aware of the potential adverse reactions of most medications in relationship to pregnancy.

    a. Should the physician prescribe an antiviral medication for the patient at this time?

    b. What antiviral would mostly likely be recommended for genital herpes if the answer to the first question is yes?

    c. What two major adverse effects are known to be associated with this drug?

CHAPTER 37

DRUGS FOR NEOPLASIA

FILL IN THE BLANK

From the textbook, find the correct word(s) to complete the statement(s).

1. Treatment strategies found to increase the effectiveness of anticancer drugs include _____ and _____.

2. Bone marrow suppression is a major adverse effect of a class of antineoplastic drugs called _____ _____.

3. By blocking the synthesis of _____ _____, methotrexate (Rheumatrex, Trexall) inhibits replication in rapidly dividing cancer cells.

4. Most antitumor antibiotics are administered _____ or through direct instillation into a body cavity using a catheter.

5. Vinca alkaloids, taxoids, and topoisomerase inhibitors are classified as _____ _____.

6. The class of antineoplastic medications referred to as _____ and _____ antagonists have fewer cytotoxic effects than seen with other antitumor medications.

7. _____ _____ modifiers assist in limiting the severe immunosuppressive effects of other anticancer drugs by stimulating the body's immune system.

Adams/Holland, *Student Workbook and Resource Guide for Pharmacology for Nurses* 4th Edition

MATCHING

For questions 8 through 13, match the type of tumor in column I with its location in the body in column II.

Column I	Column II
8. _____ adenoma	a. lymphatic tissue
9. _____ lipoma	b. central nervous system
10. _____ leukemia	c. bone, muscle, and cartilage
11. _____ lymphoma	d. glandular tissue
12. _____ glioma	e. adipose tissue
13. _____ sarcoma	f. skin
	g. blood-forming cells in bone marrow

For questions 14 through 22, match the medication in column I with its pharmacologic category in column II.

Column I	Column II
14. _____ cyclophosphamide (Cytoxan)	a. alkylating agents
15. _____ fluorouracil (5-FU, Adrucil)	b. antimetabolites
16. _____ vincristine (Oncovin)	c. antitumor antibiotics
17. _____ methotrexate (Rheumatrex, Trexall)	d. hormones and hormone antagonists
18. _____ bleomycin (Blenoxane)	e. natural products
19. _____ etoposide (VePesid)	f. biologic response modifiers and miscellaneous
20. _____ tamoxifen (Nolvadex)	
21. _____ levamisole (Ergamisol)	
22. _____ streptozocin (Zanosar)	

MULTIPLE CHOICE

23. What is the mechanism of action of antimetabolites in the treatment of neoplasia?

    a. Changing the structure of DNA in cancer cells

    b. Disrupting critical cell pathways in cancer cells

    c. Preventing cell division

    d. Activating the body's immune system

24. The nurse should instruct the patient to implement which lifestyle changes to reduce the probability of acquiring cancer?

    a. Examining the skin for abnormal lesions or changes to moles

    b. Exercising regularly and keeping body weight within normal guidelines

    c. Examining the body monthly for abnormal lumps

    d. All of the above

25. Which food(s) are NOT considered to exert protective effects against cancer?

    a. Coldwater fish

    b. Fresh fruits and vegetables

    c. Olive oil

    d. Grains and cereals

26. Which approach has a goal of eliminating 100% of cancer cells and reducing toxicity?

    a. Using multiple drugs in lower doses from different antineoplastic classes

    b. Increasing the concentration of different antineoplastic drugs

    c. Increasing the dose of one type of antineoplastic drug

    d. Combining radiation therapy with chemotherapy treatment

27. Which problem is NOT an expected adverse effect of chemotherapy?

    a. Alopecia

    b. Nausea

    c. Hypercholesterolemia

    d. Leukopenia

28. Which drug acts by altering the shape of DNA, thus preventing it from functioning normally?

    a. Cyclophosphamide (Cytoxan)

    b. Methotrexate (Rheumatrex, Trexall)

    c. Doxorubicin (Adriamycin)

    d. Vincristine (Oncovin)

29. Which is a primary drug used to treat AIDS-related Kaposi's sarcoma?

    a. Mechlorethamine (Mustargen)

    b. Floxuridine (FUDR)

    c. Doxorubicin (Adriamycin)

    d. Teniposide (Vumon)

30. Which drug is a natural product obtained from the Pacific yew plant?

    a. Mercaptopurine (6-MP, Purinethol)

    b. Paclitaxel (Taxol)

    c. Vinblastine sulfate (Velban)

    d. Flutamide (Eulexin)

31. The nurse administering vincristine (Oncovin) should monitor for which serious adverse effect?

    a. Flulike symptoms

    b. Hepatotoxicity

    c. Neurotoxicity

    d. Immunosuppression

32. Which is a preferred drug for treating breast cancer?

    a. Carboplatin (Paraplatin)

    b. Pentostatin (Nipent)

    c. Epirubicin (Ellence)

    d. Tamoxifen (Nolvadex)

33. Which anticancer drug has a similar chemical structure to the insecticide DDT?

    a. Interferon alfa-2 (Roferon-A, Intron A)

    b. Mitotane (Lysodren)

    c. Paclitaxel (Taxol)

    d. Irinotecan (Camptosar)

34. Which drug might be given for palliation of cancer in the advanced stages?

    a. Epirubicin (Ellence)

    b. Dacarbazine (DTIC-Dome)

    c. Ethinyl estradiol (Estinyl)

    d. Chlorambucil (Leukeran)

35. Which drug would NOT be used in the treatment of prostate cancer?

    a. Vinorelbine (Navelbine)

    b. Megestrol (Megace)

    c. Bicalutamide (Casodex)

    d. Leuprolide (Lupron)

36. Which drug most likely would be used for palliative treatment of malignant melanoma?

    a. Teniposide (Vumon)

    b. Idarubicin (Idamycin)

    c. Dactinomycin (Actinomycin-D, Cosmegen)

    d. Hydroxyurea (Hydrea)

37. Which drug class would most likely displace an antineoplastic drug from protein-binding sites in the plasma, increasing its effect?

    a. NSAIDs

    b. Sedative–hypnotics

    c. Antidepressants

    d. Calcium channel blockers

MAKING CONNECTIONS

38. Heart failure is sometimes observed with antineoplastic drugs. Which symptoms would be observed in a patient with heart failure?

   a. Hypokalemia

   b. Peripheral edema

   c. Dehydration

   d. Dysrhythmias

39. What are glycoprotein IIb/IIIa inhibitors used to treat?

   a. Blood coagulation disorders

   b. Depression

   c. Tuberculosis

   d. HIV-AIDS

40. Valproic acid (Depakote) is used in the pharmacotherapy of migraines, bipolar disorder, and which of the following?

   a. Schizophrenia

   b. Angina

   c. Dysrhythmias

   d. Seizures

41. Indomethacin (Indocin) is a medication that prevents prostaglandin synthesis. It is most commonly used in the treatment of which of the following?

   a. Fungal infections

   b. Pain and inflammation

   c. Hypotension

   d. Alzheimer's disease

42. The purpose for administering filgrastim (Neupogen) to patients with a sarcoma is to:

   a. boost platelet production.

   b. prevent anemia.

   c. suppress a hyperresponse of the immune system.

   d. boost neutrophil production.

CALCULATIONS

43. A patient is to receive tamoxifen 20 mg daily for the treatment of metastatic breast cancer. The medication is only available in 10-mg form. How many tablets would the patient receive per dose?

44. A patient has begun to experience periods of nausea and vomiting as an adverse reaction to the tamoxifen therapy. The order reads chlorpromazine (Compazine) 25 mg IM every 6 h prn for nausea and/or vomiting. The pharmacy has only Compazine 50 mg/2 mL available. How many milliliters should the patient receive total per day?

CASE STUDY APPLICATIONS

45. A male 40-year-old factory worker with a 10th grade education has early cancer of the prostate. He has been told that a drug killing 99% of tumor cells would be considered a very effective drug, but the remaining cells could cause his tumor to return. The patient displays lack of understanding about his condition. The nurse assigned to his patient education assesses the situation and determines the information to include in the following areas.

   a. Explain the treatment to prevent reoccurrence of the tumor in relationship to the stage of the tumor when the treatment began.

   b. Explain why classes of antineoplastics might be more effective than others in relationship to the cancer's stage.

   c. Explain the rationale for specific dosing schedules.

46. A female patient has been receiving chemotherapy for 3 weeks and has experienced a number of adverse effects including nausea, vomiting, infections, and anorexia. She is an independent 67-year-old who chooses to remain at home alone during her treatment. The home health nurse assigned to this case examines possible interventions to implement.

   a. What medications may be used to treat nausea and vomiting related to chemotherapy?

   b. What interventions may be used to lower the risk for infections?

   c. Describe the interventions for maintaining nutritional balance during chemotherapy.

47. A 32-year-old schoolteacher who recently began taking tamoxifen for metastatic breast cancer has experienced a "tumor flare." She is concerned with the outcome of this development in regard to her recovery. The nurse assigned to her examines the patient education goals and interventions.

   a. Explain this condition in regard to the medication.

   b. Explain the classification of this drug.

   c. Explain the type of tumors this medication is effective against.

   d. Explain the unique feature of this medication.

   e. Should this medication be given during pregnancy?

CHAPTER 38

DRUGS FOR ALLERGIC RHINITIS AND THE COMMON COLD

FILL IN THE BLANK

From the textbook, find the correct word(s) to complete the statement(s).

1. The fundamental problem of allergic rhinitis is inflammation of the _____ _____ of the nose, throat, and airway.

2. Drug classes used to prevent allergic rhinitis include _____, _____ _____, and _____ _____.

3. Because the sympathomimetics only relieve nasal congestion, they are often combined with _____ to control the sneezing and tearing of allergic rhinitis.

4. Oral and intranasal _____ are effective at relieving nasal congestion due to the common cold.

5. The most commonly used over-the-counter (OTC) antitussive is _____.

Adams/Holland, *Student Workbook and Resource Guide for Pharmacology for Nurses* 4th Edition

MATCHING

For questions 6 through 15, match the drug in column I with its primary class in column II.

Column I	Column II
6. _____ azelastine (Astelin)	a. H_1-receptor antagonist (antinistamine)
7. _____ oxymetazoline (Afrin 12 hr)	b. sympathomimetic
8. _____ mometasone (Nasonex)	c. intranasal corticosteroid
9. _____ diphenhydramine (Benadryl)	
10. _____ phenylephrine (Afrin-4–6 hr)	
11. _____ flunisolide (Nasalide)	
12. _____ brompheniramine (Dimetapp)	
13. _____ clemastine (Tavist)	
14. _____ beclomethasone (Beconase AQ)	
15. _____ pseudoephedrine (Sudafed)	

For questions 16 through 19, match the description in column I with its drug in column II.

Column I	Column II
16. _____ used to directly loosen thick, viscous bronchial secretions	a. benzonatate (Tessalon)
17. _____ most effective over-the-counter expectorant	b. guaifenesin (Mucinex, others)
18. _____ nonopiate antitussive having few side effects	c. dextromethorphan (Robitussin, others)
19. _____ nonopiate that acts by anesthetizing stretch receptors in the lung	d. acetylcysteine (Mucomyst)

MULTIPLE CHOICE

20. The classifications for H_1-receptor antagonists are based on the degree to which the drugs:

    a. block stomach acid secretion.

    b. affect blood coagulation.

    c. cause xerostomia.

    d. cause drowsiness.

21. In the treatment of allergies, why are newer antihistamines an improvement over the older, more traditional antihistamines?

    a. Less sedating

    b. More efficacious

    c. More potent

    d. Less GI irritation

22. Symptoms of motion sickness are often alleviated by treatment with drugs from which class?

    a. H_1-receptor antagonists

    b. H_2-receptor antagonists

    c. Immunosuppressants

    d. Intranasal corticosteroids

23. Which drug is frequently used in conjunction with analgesics and decongestants for treating the common cold?

    a. Fluticasone (Flonase)

    b. Fexofenadine (Allegra)

    c. Diphenhydramine (Benadryl)

    d. Prednisone (Meticorten)

24. Which is the most common adverse effect from therapy with diphenhydramine?

    a. Urinary retention

    b. Dysrhythmia

    c. Drowsiness

    d. Bradycardia

25. Which of the following is the most frequently reported adverse effect for intranasal corticosteroids?

    a. Sinus congestion

    b. Tachycardia

    c. Burning sensation in the nose

    d. Dry mouth

26. Which autonomic drug class is commonly used to dry the nasal mucosa?

    a. Sympathomimetics

    b. Anticholinergics

    c. Cholinergics

    d. Beta-adrenergic blockers

27. In addition to its use in reducing allergy symptoms, what is diphenhydramine (Benadryl) occasionally used to treat?

    a. Mild to moderate pain

    b. Parkinson's disease

    c. Depression

    d. Attention-deficit hyperactivity disorder

28. What is the primary action of an antitussive?

    a. Suppress the cough reflex

    b. Dry bronchial secretions

    c. Block histamine release

    d. Reduce the viscosity of bronchial secretions

29. What is the primary action of an expectorant?

    a. Suppress the cough reflex

    b. Dry bronchial secretions

    c. Reduce inflammation

    d. Reduce the viscosity of bronchial secretions

30. The most effective antitussives are from which drug class?

    a. Opioids

    b. Corticosteroids

    c. Beta$_2$ agonists

    d. NSAIDs

MAKING CONNECTIONS

31. Gingival hyperplasia is a common side effect of which of the following drugs for epilepsy?

    a. Valproic acid (Depakote)

    b. Phenobarbital

    c. Clonazepam (Klonopin)

    d. Phenytoin (Dilantin)

32. Quinapril (Accupril) lowers blood pressure by:

    a. direct dilation of arterioles.

    b. decreasing sympathetic output from the CNS.

    c. blocking the conversion of angiotensin I to angiotensin II.

    d. blocking the flow of calcium into arterioles.

33. Drugs such as epinephrine that increase the force of myocardial contraction are said to have what kind of effect?

    a. Positive inotropic

    b. Positive chronotropic

    c. Negative inotropic

    d. Negative chronotropic

34. Which of the following drugs has analgesic, anti-inflammatory, and antipyretic activity?

    a. Morphine sulfate

    b. Aspirin

    c. Acetaminophen

    d. Vicodin (hydrocodone with acetaminophen)

35. Why has the use of penicillin G declined over the past decade?

    a. There are less expensive alternatives.

    b. More people are becoming allergic to the drug.

    c. Other antibiotics are available that cause fewer side effects.

    d. Widespread microbial resistance has developed.

CALCULATIONS

36. The nurse is preparing to administer an oral suspension of acetaminophen to an infant weighing 15 kg. The order is for 10 mg/kg every 4 h. How many milligrams should the nurse administer per dose?

37. The nurse is preparing to administer an oral solution of an NSAID that contains 12.5 mg per 5 mL. The order calls for 30 mg. How many milliliters should the nurse administer?

CASE STUDY APPLICATIONS

38. A female patient comes to a clinic with history of a cold. She has been self-medicating with acetaminophen (Tylenol), diphenhydramine (Benadryl), and pseudoephedrine (Sudafed). The patient now presents with an earache and a nonproductive cough and wheezing. The health care provider prescribes Robitussin AC and a Proventil inhaler. The provider tells the patient to continue to take pseudoephedrine and acetaminophen. The provider also prescribes an antibiotic for her ear infection. The patient asks the nurse why she cannot take diphenhydramine and why the provider's choice of medications would be better than hers.

    a. What nursing diagnosis would the nurse choose for the patient?

    b. Which interventions would the nurse need to complete for the patient?

    c. What teaching should the nurse provide for each of the medications prescribed?

CHAPTER 39

DRUGS FOR ASTHMA AND OTHER PULMONARY DISORDERS

FILL IN THE BLANK

From the textbook, find the correct word(s) to complete the statement(s).

1. The two main physiologic processes of the respiratory system are _____ and _____.

2. A machine that vaporizes a liquid drug into a fine mist that can be inhaled is called a _____.

3. The two primary disorders classified as chronic obstructive pulmonary disease (COPD) are _____ and _____ _____.

4. The process of gas exchange is called _____.

5. The respiratory rate, which is normally _____ breaths per minute, can be modified by factors such as _____, _____, _____, and _____.

6. Stimulation of the parasympathetic nervous system results in _____ of the bronchioles.

7. A _____ _____ _____ device uses a propellant to deliver a measured dose of drug to the lung during each breath.

8. _____ _____ is a severe, prolonged form of asthma that is unresponsive to drug therapy and may lead to respiratory failure.

9. Goals of drug therapy for asthma are twofold: to _____ acute bronchospasm and to reduce the _____ of asthma attacks.

Adams/Holland, *Student Workbook and Resource Guide for Pharmacology for Nurses* 4th Edition
© 2014 by Pearson Education, Inc.

MATCHING

For questions 10 through 18, match the drug in column I with its primary class in column II.

Column I	Column II
10. _____ triamcinolone (Azmacort)	a. short-acting beta-adrenergic agonist
11. _____ pirbuterol (Maxair)	b. long-acting beta-adrenergic agonist
12. _____ montelukast (Singulair)	c. methylxanthine
13. _____ cromolyn (Intal)	d. anticholinergic
14. _____ budesonide (Pulmicort)	e. corticosteroid
15. _____ salmeterol (Serevent)	f. leukotriene modifier
16. _____ ipratropium (Atrovent)	g. mast cell stabilizer
17. _____ aminophylline (Truphylline)	
18. _____ fluticasone (Flovent)	

MULTIPLE CHOICE

19. During inspiration, air leaving the trachea next enters which area of the respiratory tree?

    a. Pharynx

    b. Bronchioles

    c. Alveoli

    d. Bronchi

20. Exchange of gases occurs in which pulmonary structure?

    a. Pharynx

    b. Bronchioles

    c. Alveoli

    d. Bronchi

21. When assessing a patient, the nurse must know that which of the following is NOT characteristic of asthma?

    a. Inflammation

    b. Infection

    c. Bronchoconstriction

    d. Dyspnea

22. Which of the following classes is not prescribed for asthma?

    a. Beta$_2$ agonists

    b. Methylxanthines

    c. Corticosteroids

    d. Beta blockers

23. Which of the following drug classes is most effective for relieving acute bronchospasm?

   a. Beta$_2$ agonists

   b. Mast cell stabilizers

   c. Methylxanthines

   d. Anticholinergics

24. The nurse should teach the patient that salmeterol (Serevent) is NOT indicated for the termination of acute bronchospasm for which of the following reasons?

   a. It is not absorbed orally.

   b. It takes too long to act.

   c. It affects only beta$_1$ receptors.

   d. It causes too much CNS stimulation.

25. When administering corticosteroids for the prophylaxis of nonpersistent asthma, the nurse should know that these drugs are most commonly administered by which route?

   a. Oral

   b. Topical

   c. Intranasal

   d. Intradermal

26. Corticosteroids improve asthma symptoms by which of the following mechanisms?

   a. Causing bronchodilation

   b. Suppressing inflammation

   c. Blocking histamine release

   d. Drying bronchial secretions

27. The nurse should teach the patient that long-term treatment with oral corticosteroids may cause which serious adverse effect?

   a. Rebound congestion

   b. Hypertension

   c. Cancer

   d. Adrenal atrophy

28. The nurse should know that candidiasis of the throat is a common complication during therapy with which class of medications?

   a. Inhaled corticosteroids

   b. Mast cell stabilizers

   c. Beta$_2$ agonists

   d. Mucolytics

29. The nurse should teach patients that the primary use of mast cell inhibitors in the treatment of asthma is which of the following?

   a. To terminate acute asthmatic attacks

   b. To prevent asthmatic attacks

c. To reduce secretions

d. To reduce infections

30. Nedocromil (Tilade) and cromolyn (Intal) act by which of the following mechanisms?

    a. Causing bronchodilation

    b. Suppressing the cough reflex

    c. Blocking histamine release

    d. Drying bronchial secretions

31. Patients taking zafirlukast (Accolate) or montelukast (Singulair) should be taught that they will see improvement within what time frame?

    a. 2 hours

    b. 2 days

    c. 1 week

    d. 1 month

32. What is the most common reason for school absenteeism?

    a. Asthma

    b. Ear infections

    c. Colds

    d. Heart disease

33. Why are selective beta$_1$-agonists ineffective for treating asthma?

    a. There are no beta$_1$ receptors in bronchial smooth muscle.

    b. They cannot be delivered by the inhalation route.

    c. They cause bronchoconstriction.

    d. Their duration of action is too short.

MAKING CONNECTIONS

34. Trizivir is a combination drug that contains abacavir, lamivudine, and zidovudine. This drug is used to treat which infection?

    a. Bacterial

    b. Fungal

    c. Herpes

    d. HIV-AIDS

35. The nurse would administer which of the following for opioid overdose?

    a. Methadone (Dolophine)

    b. Epinephrine (Adrenalin)

    c. Naloxone (Narcan)

    d. Dobutamine (Dobutrex)

36. Epoetin alfa (Epogen) is administered to:

    a. boost the immune system.

    b. increase the number of erythrocytes.

    c. reduce neurotoxicity of antineoplastic medications.

    d. promote passive immunity.

37. Patients taking aminoglycosides should be monitored for:

    a. nephrotoxicity.

    b. pulmonary toxicity.

    c. hypertension.

    d. dysrhythmias.

38. Cyclopentolate (Cyclogyl) is an anticholinergic. What effect would the nurse expect this drug to have on the respiratory system of an asthmatic patient?

    a. The patient will experience dyspnea.

    b. The patient will exhibit increased respiratory secretions.

    c. The patient will experience mucosal drying and increased heart rate.

    d. The patient will likely experience no effects on the respiratory system.

CALCULATIONS

39. A patient has aminophylline ordered at 0.25 mg/kg/hr. The patient weighs 50 kg. How many milligrams should be administered over a 6-hour period?

40. A patient has albuterol 4 mg ordered tid. A concentrate of 2 mg in 5 mL is available. How many milliliters would be given per each dose?

CASE STUDY APPLICATIONS

41. A male has been admitted to a respiratory unit after being treated in the emergency department (ED) for an exacerbation of asthma. The patient states he has been on beclomethasone (Beconase) inhaler and an oral theophylline preparation for about 2 months. His last exacerbation of asthma was about 2 months ago, and he claims to be compliant with his medications. About a week ago, the patient started having a persistent cough, productive of green thick sputum. He has been short of breath and has been wheezing in the ED. The physician prescribes lorazepam (Ativan) and metaproterenol (Alupent) while the patient is in the ED. The nurse has chosen a nursing diagnosis of *Ineffective Airway Clearance* due to an infection process causing increased mucus production.

    a. Which assessment would indicate a possible infection and ineffective airway clearance?

    b. Which nursing interventions would need to be completed for the diagnosis of *Ineffective Airway Clearance*?

    c. Give the therapeutic rationales for the two drugs taken by the patient prior to the ED visit.

    d. Give the therapeutic rationales for the two drugs taken by the patient during his ED visit.

CHAPTER 40

DRUGS FOR PEPTIC ULCER DISEASE

FILL IN THE BLANK

From the textbook, find the correct word(s) to complete the statement(s).

1. The digestive system consists of two basic anatomical divisions: the _____ canal and the _____ organs.

2. The primary functions of the GI tract are to physically _____ ingested food and to provide the necessary _____ and surface area for chemical _____ and _____ of nutrients into the bloodstream.

3. The small intestine is lined with tiny projections called _____ and _____ that provide a huge surface area for the absorption of food and _____.

4. Substances are propelled along the GI tract by the process of _____, rhythmic contraction of layers of _____ muscle.

5. The _____ _____ prevents the stomach contents from moving backwards into the esophagus and causing a condition known as _____ _____.

6. The _____ cells secrete pepsinogen and the _____ cells secrete hydrochloric acid and _____ _____, which are essential for the absorption of vitamin B_{12}.

7. Gastric juice is the most _____ in the body and has a pH of _____.

8. External risk factors associated with peptic ulcer disease (PUD) include drugs, particularly _____, _____, and _____.

9. The primary cause of PUD is infection by the gram-negative bacterium _____ _____.

MATCHING

For questions 10 through 15, match the correct term in column I with the definition in column II.

Column I	Column II
10. _____ GERD	a. ulcerations in the lower small intestine
11. _____ PUD	b. hypersecretion of gastric acid
12. _____ Crohn's disease	c. lesion located in the stomach or small intestine
13. _____ ulcerative colitis	d. increased acid secretion in the stomach
14. _____ H₂ receptors	e. backward movement of stomach contents into the esophagus
15. _____ Zollinger-Ellison syndrome	f. erosions located in the large intestine

MULTIPLE CHOICE

16. For a patient taking high doses of aluminum hydroxide, the nurse should assess for which frequent adverse effect?

    a. Constipation

    b. GERD

    c. Diarrhea

    d. Muscle pain

17. The nurse should understand that omeprazole (Prilosec) acts to reduce symptoms of PUD by what mechanism?

    a. Neutralizing stomach acid

    b. Inhibiting secretion of gastric acid

    c. Eliminating *H. pylori*

    d. Slowing peristalsis in the upper GI tract

18. In caring for a patient with PUD, the nurse must understand that digestive enzymes are secreted by all of the following EXCEPT:

    a. salivary glands.

    b. stomach.

    c. pancreas.

    d. microvilli.

19. The nurse is developing education materials for a pregnant patient. Which of the following nonpharmacologic therapies should be recommended?

    a. St. John's wort

    b. Black cohosh

    c. Valerian

    d. Ginger

20. During an assessment, the nurse should recognize which characteristic symptom as most indicative of a duodenal ulcer?

    a. Gnawing pain or burning in the upper abdomen

    b. Nighttime pain, nausea, and vomiting

    c. Bright red blood in the stool

    d. Bright red blood in vomit

21. The patient has a prior history of gastric ulcers. Which of the following would be increased in the presence of a recurrence?

    a. Hunger, even after meals

    b. Frequency of remissions

    c. Frequency in 30- to 50-year-old age group

    d. Pain, briefly relieved by food

22. Inflammatory bowel disease (IBD) includes which of the following?

    a. Both gastric and duodenal ulcers

    b. Zollinger-Ellison syndrome

    c. Crohn's disease and ulcerative colitis

    d. PUD and GERD

23. The patient is overweight and complaining of an intense burning (heartburn) in the chest, which is indicative of which of the following conditions?

    a. PUD

    b. GERD

    c. IBD

    d. Crohn's disease

24. In developing a plan of care for the patient with PUD, the nurse needs to include all of the following EXCEPT:

    a. smoking cessation.

    b. abstinence from alcohol.

    c. avoidance of caffeine.

    d. severe dietary restrictions.

25. Which class of drugs reduces acid secretion in the stomach by binding irreversibly to an enzyme on the parietal cells?

    a. H_2-receptor antagonists

    b. Serotonin receptor antagonists

    c. Proton pump inhibitors

    d. Antacids

26. Which class of peptic ulcer medications consists of alkaline combinations of aluminum hydroxide and magnesium hydroxide?

    a. Phenothiazines

    b. Serotonin receptor antagonists

    c. Proton pump inhibitors

    d. Antacids

27. Which of the following best describes the mechanism of action of sucralfate (Carafate)?

    a. Kills *H. pylori*

    b. Adds a gel-like protective mucus over the ulcer

    c. Reduces secretion of acid

    d. Increases the secretion of bicarbonate

MAKING CONNECTIONS

28. Why is tetracycline not used in children under 12 years of age?

    a. Causes penicillin-like reactions

    b. Stains deciduous teeth

    c. Is primarily used to treat acne

    d. Only used to treat Lyme disease

29. Why is clarithromycin (Biaxin) effective against *H. pylori*?

    a. It is effective against gram-positive and gram-negative organisms.

    b. It is a macrolide that can be given to people with penicillin allergies.

    c. It is considered to be a broad-spectrum antibiotic.

    d. All of the above are true.

30. All of the following are true about metronidazole (Flagyl) EXCEPT:

    a. it is considered an antibacterial agent.

    b. it is effective in the treatment of STDs.

    c. it is classified as an aminoglycoside.

    d. it is used in the treatment of protozoal infections.

31. A female patient is prescribed oral albuterol (Proventil) for asthma. Which of the following administration instructions should the nurse give?

    a. Always take the medication with food.

    b. Do not take this medication to terminate acute asthma attacks.

    c. Remain upright for at least 30 minutes after taking the medication.

    d. Take the medication at night to avoid drowsiness.

32. A male patient is receiving an HMG-CoA reductase inhibitor. He is most likely being treated for which of the following?

    a. High lipid levels in the blood

    b. Stroke

    c. Schizophrenia

    d. Hypertension

CALCULATIONS

33. The patient is to receive the following medication: ranitidine (Zantac) 50 mg IV in 100 mL to infuse in 30 min by microdrip. Calculate the correct dosages as required.

    a. How many gtt per hour is this?

    b. How many milliliters per hour will the nurse set the infusion pump to deliver?

34. The patient is to receive the following medication: aluminum hydroxide (Amphojel) 2 T qid PO.

    a. What times would the nurse give this medication?

    b. Provide the correct equivalents in teaspoons, milliliters, and ounces.

CASE STUDY APPLICATIONS

35. An elderly male is admitted with a recurrence of gastric ulcers. His wife tells you that he has been taking cimetidine (Tagamet) as an OTC preparation. She tells you that he no longer complains of the gnawing pain in his stomach but has become increasingly confused within the past 3 days. During the nurse's initial assessment, the nurse notes that the patient is oriented to person and time but not place.

    a. Name at least two appropriate nursing diagnoses for this patient.

    b. Prioritize the diagnoses and provide rationales.

36. The nurse continues to care for the patient described in question 35. The nurse notes that cimetidine has been discontinued by the health care provider's order. The patient is now on ranitidine (Zantac).

    a. What would be the nurse's short-term goal for this patient?

    b. During the implementation of the plan for care, what laboratory values would the nurse assess for this patient? Why?

37. While the nurse is preparing the patient described in question 35 for discharge, he has been placed on omeprazole (Prilosec) and antacids. In preparing the patient education for both the patient and his wife related to these medications, answer the following questions.

    a. What would be an appropriate nursing diagnosis for this couple?

    b. What basic instruction is necessary in relation to OTC medications?

    c. What does this patient need to know about the timing of his medications?

CHAPTER 41

DRUGS FOR BOWEL DISORDERS AND OTHER GASTROINTESTINAL CONDITIONS

FILL IN THE BLANK

From the textbook, find the correct word(s) to complete the statement(s).

1. Psychological factors related to nausea occur during periods of extreme _____ or when confronted with unpleasant _____, _____, and _____.

2. The two major drug classes used to effectively treat nausea due to motion sickness are _____ and _____.

3. Ingestion of poisons is sometimes treated by administering _____ such as _____ to induce _____ within 15 minutes.

4. _____ are used for the treatment of obesity, although they produce only _____ effects.

5. Constipation is identified by a decrease in the _____ and number of _____ _____.

6. The etiology of constipation may be related to insufficient _____ _____, especially insoluble _____ _____.

7. Severe constipation can lead to a fecal _____ and a complete _____ of the bowel.

8. Prophylactic pharmacotherapy with a _____ is appropriate to preclude straining or bearing down during _____.

Adams/Holland, *Student Workbook and Resource Guide for Pharmacology for Nurses* 4th Edition
© 2014 by Pearson Education, Inc.

9. The role of the nurse in the pharmacotherapy of bowel disorders involves careful _____ of a patient's condition and providing _____.

10. Laxatives are contraindicated in _____ _____, _____ _____, and _____ _____because of the risk for causing bowel perforation.

MATCHING

For questions 11 through 17, match the correct term in column I with the definition in column II.

Column I	Column II
11. _____ laxative	a. causes water and fat to be absorbed into stools
12. _____ cathartic	b. promotes defecation
13. _____ bulk-forming agent	c. lubricates the stool and colon
14. _____ stool softener	d. irritates the bowel, causing peristalsis
15. _____ stimulant	e. absorbs water, increasing size of fecal mass
16. _____ osmotic	f. pulls water into stool for a more watery stool
17. _____ mineral oil	g. implies a strong and complete bowel emptying

MULTIPLE CHOICE

18. Which of the following patient complaints would cause the nurse to discontinue laxative therapy?

    a. Nausea with dry skin

    b. Mild abdominal discomfort

    c. Diarrhea and cramping

    d. A soft-formed stool

19. All of the following describe stimulant laxatives EXCEPT:

    a. peristalsis is increased by irritating the colon.

    b. results are both rapid and effective.

    c. never used in combination with other types.

    d. frequently used as an aid in bowel preparation.

20. Patients receiving prochlorperazine (Compazine) for nausea must also be monitored for which of the following?

    a. Extrapyramidal symptoms

    b. Cholinergic side effects

    c. Early Parkinson's disease

    d. Hyperemesis gravidarum

21. Patient education for laxative therapy should include which of the following?

    a. Goals of therapy

    b. Reason for treatment

    c. Possible adverse effects

    d. All of the above

22. A nursing assessment of a patient on laxative therapy should include all of the following EXCEPT:

    a. vital signs.

    b. abdominal assessment.

    c. level of consciousness.

    d. character of stool.

23. Which of the following is a bulk-forming laxative?

    a. Psyllium mucilloid (Metamucil)

    b. Docusate (Colace)

    c. Senna root

    d. *Cascara sagrada*

24. Aprepitant (Emend) is a newer antiemetic that belongs to which of the following drug classifications?

    a. Neurokinin receptors

    b. Serotonin-receptor blockers

    c. Glucocorticoids

    d. Phenothiazines

25. The nurse should recognize which of the following as a potential complication secondary to the administration of bulk-forming laxatives?

    a. Bowel perforation

    b. Severe hypotension

    c. Stimulation of defecation

    d. Obstruction of the esophagus

26. Which of the following categories of laxatives have a high sodium content?

    a. Bulk-forming laxatives

    b. Stimulant laxatives

    c. Osmotic laxatives

    d. Herbal laxative preparations

27. Which of the following drugs is a first-line drug for the control of inflammatory bowel disease?

    a. Prochlorperazine (Compazine)

    b. Sulfasalazine (Azulfidine)

    c. Loperamide (Imodium)

    d. Dimenhydrinate (Dramamine)

28. The health care provider has ordered pancrelipase, 10000 units bid. The nurse should know that this drug should be administered:

    a. just prior to a meal.

    b. before bedtime.

    c. with as little liquid as possible.

    d. with milk or an antacid.

29. Scopolamine (Transderm-Scop) is an effective antiemetic for motion sickness that is classified as a(n):

    a. adrenergic agonist.

    b. cholinergic agonist.

    c. anticholinergic.

    d. ganglionic blocker.

MAKING CONNECTIONS

30. Dyphylline is a xanthine drug similar to theophylline; it relaxes smooth muscle. What is its primary indication?

    a. Shock

    b. Asthma

    c. Parkinson's disease

    d. Migraines

31. Diphenhydramine (Benadryl) is an antihistamine. Which of the following is an expected adverse effect?

    a. Headache

    b. Nasal stuffiness

    c. Drowsiness

    d. Salivation

32. Indapamide (Lozol) is a thiazide-like diuretic that is chemically related to sulfonamides. What are many sulfonamides used to treat?

    a. Peptic ulcers

    b. Viral infections

    c. Bacterial infections

    d. Anxiety

33. Naldecon Senior DX is a combination drug consisting of dextromethorphan 10 mg and guaifenesin 200 mg. Naldecon is most likely prescribed for which of the following?

    a. Cold and flu symptoms

    b. Mild to moderate pain

    c. Asthma

    d. Hypertension

34. Alkylating agents such as cyclophosphamide (Cytoxan) are primarily used to treat which of the following?

    a. Asthma

    b. Bipolar disorder

    c. Cancer

    d. HIV-AIDS

CALCULATIONS

35. The patient is to receive prochlorperazine (Compazine) 10 mg every 4–6 h IM prn for relief of nausea and vomiting. The medication on hand is 25 mg per 2-mL ampule.

    a. How much of this medication will be used for each dose?

    b. What type of syringe should be used?

    c. What length and gauge needle is appropriate for this medication?

36. To control loose stools, the patient has been prescribed diphenoxylate with atropine (Lomotil). A dose of 2.5 mg PO qid has been ordered. How many milligrams will this patient receive in 24 hours?

CASE STUDY APPLICATIONS

37. A male is admitted complaining of an inability to move his bowels for the past 5 days. The nurse observes that his abdomen is distended; he is somewhat anxious; and his vital signs are slightly elevated in comparison to those received in a report from the emergency department (ED) nurse. The health care provider has ordered an osmotic laxative.

    a. Identify two high-priority nursing diagnoses for this patient.

    b. What are the goals related to each of these diagnoses?

    c. List at least two nursing actions that will be implemented to assist in achieving these goals.

    d. What criteria would the nurse use to determine the effectiveness of the plan of care based on patient outcomes?

38. An 82-year-old female patient complains of diarrhea for the past 3 days. She states she has had five or more liquefied stools a day during this time. She has not noted any bleeding, however. Antidiarrheal therapy has begun.

    a. What will the nurse include in the initial assessment?

    b. What objective data will be important for the nurse to observe?

    c. What safety issues need to be considered?

39. A 24-year-old female patient is admitted with severe nausea and vomiting. She tells the nurse that she has experienced this discomfort every morning for a week. Her pregnancy test comes back positive. This condition is known as hyperemesis gravidarum. Intravenous fluids are ordered along with an antiemetic.

    a. What assessment will the nurse make to ensure the safety of mother and fetus?

    b. What is the primary therapeutic goal for this patient?

    c. Prochlorperazine (Compazine) is the prototype drug of antiemetics. Would it be appropriate for this patient? If not, why?

    d. What outcome criteria will alert the nurse to the fact that this patient's goals have been accomplished?

40. The nurse assists with the admission of a female patient who is 350 lb, 5 ft 8 in. She is complaining of hunger, stating, "I have not eaten since yesterday." It is now noontime and dinner trays are being served. The patient tells the nurse that she is not only "hungry" but has a "large appetite" and requests two cheeseburgers for lunch instead of the usual one that appears on her tray. The nurse notes on her admission assessment that she has been on the anorexiant orlistat (Xenical).

   a. What dietary restrictions should be part of this patient's education?

   b. What supplemental medications may be needed because of the decreased absorption of other substances?

   c. What nonpharmacologic support will supplement the care plan of this patient in relation to her "hunger," "appetite," and "weight reduction program"?

CHAPTER 42

DRUGS FOR NUTRITIONAL DISORDERS

FILL IN THE BLANK

From the textbook, find the correct word(s) to complete the statement(s).

1. Vitamins are _____ _____ required by the body in small amounts for _____ and for the maintenance of _____ _____ _____.

2. An important characteristic of vitamins is that, with the exception of vitamin _____, human cells cannot _____ them.

3. Without vitamin K, abnormal _____ is produced and _____ _____ is affected.

4. Vitamins that dissolve in lipids are called _____ _____ and include vitamins _____, _____, _____, and _____.

5. _____ vitamins cannot be absorbed in the _____ _____ but can be stored in large quantities in the _____ and adipose tissue.

6. Recommended _____ _____ values represent the _____ amount of vitamin or mineral needed to prevent a _____ in a healthy adult.

7. _____, or toxic levels of vitamins, have been reported for vitamins _____, _____, _____, _____, _____, _____, and _____.

8. _____ _____ is the most common cause of thiamine deficiency in the United States.

Adams/Holland, *Student Workbook and Resource Guide for Pharmacology for Nurses* 4th Edition
© 2014 by Pearson Education, Inc.

9. Vitamin D$_2$, also known as _____, is obtained from fortified milk, margarine, and other dairy products.

10. _____ _____ is considered a primary antioxidant, preventing the formation of _____ _____ that damage cell membranes and other cellular structures.

MATCHING

For questions 11 through 17, match the correct term in column I with the definition in column II.

Column I

11. _____ vitamin K

12. _____ vitamins A, D, E, and K

13. _____ vitamin A deficiency

14. _____ vitamin D

15. _____ vitamin B complex

16. _____ vitamin B$_6$

17. _____ vitamin B$_9$

Column II

a. problems with night vision

b. skeletal abnormalities

c. synthesis of heme

d. fat-soluble vitamins

e. antidote for warfarin (Coumadin)

f. folic acid

g. twelve different vitamins

MULTIPLE CHOICE

18. Which of the following statements does NOT refer to vitamin B$_{12}$ (cyanocobalamin)?

a. Important in cell replication

b. Lack results in pernicious anemia

c. Important in myelin synthesis

d. Deficiency results in uremia

19. Patient education related to vitamins must include which of the following statements?

a. Specific reason for prescribed vitamin therapy

b. Monitoring specific brands being taken by the patient

c. RDAs as stated on the label

d. Side effects that occur at high doses

20. Which of the following vitamins would the nurse recommend to promote immune system health and tissue healing?

a. Vitamin D (ergocalciferol)

b. Vitamin E (tocopherols)

c. Vitamin A (Aquasol)

d. Vitamin C (ascorbic acid)

21. One of the anorexiants approved for the short-term therapy of obesity, believed to act by serotonin (5-HT) receptors in the brain, causing a feeling of fullness or satiety is

    a. locaserin (Belviq)

    b. orlistat (Alli, Xenical)

    c. sibutramine (Meridia)

    d. amphetamine and dextroamphetamine (Dexedrine)

22. A patient is likely to receive total parenteral nutrition (TPN) for which of the following conditions?

    a. Major surgery

    b. Bowel obstruction

    c. Supplement oral intake

    d. Difficulty swallowing

23. Macrominerals or microminerals require patient education of which of the following?

    a. They should be taken at less than the recommended RDA.

    b. They are organic substances necessary to maintain homeostasis.

    c. They can reach toxic levels if taken in excess.

    d. Minerals are necessary for lipid lowering to occur.

24. Patient education for TPN must include which of the following?

    a. Clean technique when changing dressings and tubing

    b. Signs and symptoms of hyperglycemia

    c. Need to report increased feelings of hunger

    d. Stabilization of nutritional status

25. When the patient is on loop diuretics, the nurse will need to assess which of the following?

    a. Potassium level

    b. Sodium level

    c. Magnesium level

    d. All of the above

26. Hypomagnesemia will produce which of the following symptoms?

    a. Nausea, vomiting, and constipation

    b. Weakness, anorexia, and bleeding abnormalities

    c. Muscular twitches, cramps, and spasms

    d. General weakness, hypertension, and respiratory depression

27. Why must patients receiving TPN be monitored for fluid volume excess/overload?

    a. TPN is a hypertonic solution that can cause a fluid shift.

    b. Endogenous insulin is insufficient for glucose metabolism.

    c. Strict aseptic technique will prevent infections.

    d. Weighing will assist with monitoring intake and output.

MAKING CONNECTIONS

28. The patient complains of gnawing pain in the epigastric area that is temporarily relieved by food, but then recurs within 30 min after eating. The patient has a history of PUD. Which diagnosis should the nurse suspect?

    a. Gastric ulcer

    b. Duodenal ulcer

    c. Crohn's disease

    d. IBS

29. Diphenoxylate with atropine (Lomotil) is an opioid that is given to relieve diarrhea. Why is atropine added to this medication?

    a. To prevent abuse of this medication

    b. To dry up loose stools and secretions

    c. To provide an anticholinergic response

    d. To provide a cholinergic response

30. Psyllium mucilloid (Metamucil) is a bulk-forming drug that is used with which of the following combinations?

    a. Laxative or antidiarrheal

    b. Laxative or antiemetic

    c. Antidiarrheal or antiflatulent

    d. Antidiarrheal or antiemetic

31. Scopolamine (Transderm-Scop) is an effective antiemetic that is usually prescribed as which of the following?

    a. Liquid suspension

    b. Subcutaneous injection

    c. Transdermal patch

    d. Intramuscular injection

32. Herbal remedies for diarrhea include which of the following preparations?

    a. Senna root

    b. Cascara leaves

    c. Acidophilus

    d. Sibutramine

CALCULATIONS

33. The patient has pernicious anemia. The order reads: Administer cyanocobalamin 200 mcg/mo IM. The vial reads 100 mcg/mL in a 30-mL vial. How much will the nurse give per monthly dose?

34. The patient has hypomagnesemia. He is about to receive 250 mg in 250 mL over 4 hours. How many milliliters per hour will he receive?

CASE STUDY APPLICATIONS

35. A 78-year-old patient has developed aspiration pneumonia due to an impaired swallowing reflex. The physician has decided to place a gastroscopy tube for enteral feedings. He is to be placed on a specialized feeding. During the initial assessment, the nurse determines the following:

    a. Because of his respiratory condition, he will require a custom food supplement. Which would the nurse recommend? Why?

    b. Laboratory tests will determine his ability to heal. What laboratory results will the nurse need to monitor?

    c. Name the four types of enteral feedings that are available.

    d. What is the nurse's overall goal for this patient?

    e. What nursing interventions will the nurse employ to aid in achieving this goal?

    f. What evaluative criteria will the nurse use to determine if the goal was met?

36. A female patient had a stroke, so the nurse believes that TPN is in order. The patient goes to the operating room for the insertion of a central line. During the postop assessment, the nurse notes the solution infusing at the site of insertion.

    a. What type of solution will this patient receive?

    b. Why is this form of feeding necessary?

    c. What is the short-term goal for this patient?

    d. What is the long-term goal for this patient?

    e. What nursing interventions are required in this patient's care?

    f. How will the nurse evaluate the effectiveness of the plan of care?

37. A male patient is admitted with malabsorption syndrome secondary to chemotherapy. The health care provider discusses with the patient the need for central line placement for this procedure.

    a. Why is a central line necessary? What nursing diagnosis would the nurse use for this patient?

    b. Will this type of feeding be short term? What is the nurse's goal for this patient?

    c. Can the patient return home with this type of feeding?

CHAPTER 43

DRUGS FOR PITUITARY, THYROID, AND ADRENAL DISORDERS

FILL IN THE BLANK

From the textbook, find the correct word(s) to complete the statements(s).

1. _____ are chemical messengers released in response to a change in the body's internal environment.

2. When administering antidiuretic hormones, the nurse should carefully assess _____ and _____ balance.

3. Two preparations available for the treatment of diabetes insipidus are _____ and _____.

4. Prior to administration of levothyroxine (Levothroid, Synthroid, others), the nurse should thoroughly assess the patient's _____ system.

5. Graves' disease may cause tachycardia, weight loss, elevated body temperature, and _____.

6. Propylthiouracil (PTU) may cause GI distress and should be administered _____ meals.

7. The nurse must be aware that glucocorticoids increase the patient's susceptibility to _____.

Adams/Holland, *Student Workbook and Resource Guide for Pharmacology for Nurses* 4th Edition
© 2014 by Pearson Education, Inc.

MATCHING

For questions 8 through 12, match the specific disease in column I with its related concept in column II.

Column I

8. _____ Cushing's syndrome

9. _____ adrenal cortex hyposecretion

10. _____ Graves' disease

11. _____ myxedema (adults)
    and cretinism (children)

12. _____ diabetes insipidus

Column II

a. thyroid hormone (Levothroid, Synthroid, others)

b. deficiency in ADH

c. linked to glucocorticoid use

d. glucocorticoids

e. propylthiouracil (PTU)

For questions 13 through 15, match the drug in column I with its class in column II.

Column I

13. _____ prednisone

14. _____ liotrix (Thyrolar)

15. _____ methimazole (Tapazole)

Column II

a. thyroid medication

b. antithyroid medication

c. glucocorticoid

MULTIPLE CHOICE

16. The nurse is monitoring a patient's lab tests and notices a rise in parathyroid hormone (PTH). Which of the following lab values may also occur in this patient?

    a. Increased blood glucose

    b. Decreased blood glucose

    c. Decreased serum calcium

    d. Increased serum calcium

17. The nurse understands that negative feedback ensures endocrine homeostasis by doing which of the following?

    a. Stimulating the release of a secondary hormone

    b. Stimulating the release of a primary hormone

    c. Inhibiting the action of a secondary hormone

    d. Inhibiting the action of a primary hormone

18. The nurse is caring for a patient who is receiving hormone replacement therapy (HRT). Which of the following is NOT an example of HRT?

    a. Thyroid hormone after thyroidectomy

    b. Supplying insulin to a patient whose pancreas is not functioning

    c. Testosterone for breast cancer

    d. Adrenal cortex dysfunction

19. Which of the following hormones is NOT released from the anterior pituitary gland?

    a. Thyroid-stimulating hormone (TSH)

    b. Antidiuretic hormone

    c. Growth hormone

    d. Adrenocorticotropic hormone (ACTH)

20. A patient receiving levothyroxine (Levothroid, Synthroid, others) may experience which of the following adverse effects?

    a. Loss of weight

    b. Lack of energy

    c. Reduced pulse rate

    d. Reduced body temperature

21. It is important that the nurse teach female patients that long-term use of levothyroxine (Levothroid, Synthroid, others) may be associated with which of the following symptoms?

    a. Osteoporosis

    b. Decreased white blood cell count

    c. Weight gain

    d. Decreased incidence of insomnia

22. The nurse would most likely administer antithyroid medications to patients with which of the following symptoms?

    a. Dysrhythmia

    b. Weight loss

    c. Reduced activity

    d. Anemia

23. Which of the following hormones will ultimately result in release of glucocorticoids from the adrenal glands?

    a. Corticotropin releasing factor (CRF)

    b. Adrenocorticotropic hormone (ACTH)

    c. Falling levels of cortisol

    d. All of the above

24. Which of the following drugs is often administered by alternate-day dosing and requires the nurse to provide specific patient teaching?

    a. Thyroid hormone

    b. Antithyroid therapy

    c. Corticosteroids

    d. Insulin

25. In caring for a patient with Cushing's syndrome, the nurse understands this disorder is associated with which of the following hormones?

    a. Mineralocorticoids

    b. Glucocorticoids

c. Androgens

d. ADH

26. The nurse should observe for which of the following adverse effects of hydrocortisone (Cortef, others) therapy?

    a. Asthma

    b. Rhinitis

    c. Nausea

    d. Mood and personality changes

27. Which of the following corticosteroids has mineralocorticoid activity?

    a. Hydrocortisone (Cortef, others)

    b. Methylprednisolone (Dep-Medrol, Medrol, others)

    c. Prednisolone

    d. Prednisone

28. A deficiency of growth hormone will result in which of the following?

    a. Dwarfism

    b. Diabetes insipidus

    c. Urinary retention

    d. Mental impairment

29. Vasopressin is prescribed for which of the following primary symptoms?

    a. Altered metabolism

    b. Polyuria

    c. Inflammation

    d. Altered glucose blood levels

MAKING CONNECTIONS

30. Which of the following will change during thyroid therapy if only the heart rate increases?

    a. Dysrhythmia

    b. Peripheral vascular resistance

    c. Cardiac output

    d. Stroke volume

31. Cholestyramine (Questran) will decrease the absorption of levothyroxine (Levothroid, Synthroid, others) if given at the same time. Patients take cholestyramine for what type of disorders?

    a. Hypertension

    b. High blood cholesterol levels

    c. Peptic ulcers

    d. Weight gain

32. Fluconazole (Diflucan) and other azole drugs are indicated for which of the following?

    a. Fungal infections

    b. Malaria

    c. Diarrhea

    d. Constipation

33. Which vitamin is considered to be an antidote for overdoses of warfarin (Coumadin)?

    a. A

    b. B_2

    c. B_{12}

    d. K

34. A drug's trade name is assigned by which of the following?

    a. Physician

    b. Pharmacist

    c. Drug manufacturer

    d. FDA

CALCULATIONS

35. The physician ordered vasopressin 10 units SC bid for a patient. The pharmacy has vasopressin 20 units/mL. How many milliliters will the nurse administer?

36. The physician ordered propylthiouracil 200 mg PO for a patient. The pharmacy has propylthiouracil 50-mg tablets. How many tablets will the nurse administer?

CASE STUDY APPLICATIONS

37. A female patient is diabetic and is also a candidate for thyroid therapy because of her hypothyroid disorder. Examples of the medications she might take include levothyroxine sodium (Levothroid, Synthroid, others), liothyronine (Cytomel, Triostat), and liotrix (Thyrolar).

    a. In planning proper care, what complications of using these drugs simultaneously would the nurse consider?

    b. What nursing interventions would be appropriate?

38. A 35-year-old male patient is diagnosed with Graves' disease. He wants to know how his new medication propylthiouracil (PTU) will affect his life.

    a. List the important patient teaching related to PTU.

    b. Describe nursing interventions that will assist this patient in adjusting to his medication regimen.

CHAPTER 44

DRUGS FOR DIABETES MELLITUS

FILL IN THE BLANK

From the textbook, find the correct word(s) to complete the statements(s).

1. Juvenile-onset diabetes is called _____ _____ _____ _____;
   age-onset diabetes is referred to as _____ _____ _____ _____.

2. A class of drugs prescribed after diet and exercise have failed to bring blood glucose levels to within normal limits is _____ _____.

3. In type II diabetes mellitus, insulin receptors in the target tissues have become _____ to the hormone.

4. The treatment goal with insulin therapy is to maintain _____ _____ levels within strict normal limits.

Adams/Holland, *Student Workbook and Resource Guide for Pharmacology for Nurses* 4th Edition
© 2014 by Pearson Education, Inc.

MATCHING

For questions 5 through 7, match the drug therapy in column I with the specific disease in column II.

Column I	Column II
5. _____ regular insulin (Humulin R, Novolin R)	a. type I diabetes mellitus
	b. type II diabetes mellitus
6. _____ glipizide (Glucotrol)	
7. _____ tolbutamide (Orinase)	

For questions 8 through 12, match the drug in column I with its classification in column II.

Column I	Column II
8. _____ glyburide (DiaBeta, Micronase)	a. alpha-glucosidase inhibitor
9. _____ nateglinide (Starlix)	b. biguanide
10. _____ metformin immediate-release (Glucophage, Riomet)	c. meglitinide
11. _____ acarbose (Precose)	d. sulfonylurea
12. _____ pioglitazone (Actos)	e. thiazolidinedione

MULTIPLE CHOICE

13. Which of the following stimulates the pancreas to secrete insulin?

    a. Hyperglycemia

    b. Hypoglycemia

    c. Glucagon

    d. Ketoacids

14. While taking a health history, the nurse should recognize that which of the following is NOT a short-term sign of type I diabetes mellitus?

    a. Polyuria

    b. Polyphagia

    c. Acidosis

    d. Polydipsia

15. When giving insulin, the nurse knows the most common route of administration is which of the following?

    a. Oral

    b. Intradermal

    c. Subcutaneous

    d. Intramuscular

16. When planning follow-up care, the nurse should know that which of the following is a longer-acting form of insulin?

    a. Insulin lispro (Humalog)

    b. Insulin, isophane (NPH, Humulin N, Novolin N, ReliOn N)

    c. insulin glargine (Lantus)

    d. insulin aspart (NovoLog)

17. Which of the following adverse effects does the nurse recognize when too much insulin has been administered?

    a. Hypoglycemia

    b. Tachycardia

    c. Convulsions

    d. All of the above

18. When giving oral hypoglycemics, the nurse expects which of the following actions to occur?

    a. The pancreas is stimulated to secrete more insulin.

    b. Insulin receptors become more sensitive to target tissues.

    c. The liver is inhibited from releasing glucose.

    d. Both a and b

19. Persons with type I or type II diabetes who are not able to achieve glucose control by the use of insulin alone might be administered this insulin adjunct, resembling a natural hormone found in beta cells of the pancreas.

    a. Metformin (Glucophage)

    b. Pramlintide (Symlin)

    c. Novolog Mix

    d. Humalog Mix

20. During oral hypoglycemic therapy, the nurse should assess for which symptoms related to abnormalities in liver function?

    a. Yellowed skin, pale stools, dark urine

    b. Pink skin, light brown stools, yellow urine

    c. Pale skin, red-tinged stools, amber urine

    d. Red skin, dark stools, clear urine

21. If injection sites are not rotated regularly, the diabetic patient may suffer from which of the following?

    a. Petechiae

    b. Lipodystrophy

    c. Hematoma

    d. Pustules

22. Which of the following nursing diagnoses is NOT appropriate for the patient receiving insulin therapy?

    a. *Risk for Injury*

    b. *Risk for Imbalanced Nutrition*

    c. *Risk for Role Confusion*

    d. *Risk for Infection*

23. When considering glucose regulation in the body, which of the following components of homeostasis would be restored following insulin therapy?

    a. Sensor (senses glucose in the bloodstream)

    b. Control center (determines the set point for glucose levels in the bloodstream)

    c. Effector (responds to the increased levels of glucose in the bloodstream)

    d. Receptor (produces a response at the site of glucose action)

MAKING CONNECTIONS

24. If a patient is prescribed regular insulin (Humulin R, Novolin R) and is also prescribed antihypertensive drugs, which of the following would likely mask symptoms of hypoglycemic reaction due to insulin therapy?

    a. Hydrochlorothiazide (HydroDIURIL)

    b. Timolol (Betimol, others)

    c. Nifedipine (Procardia)

    d. Enalapril (Vasotec)

25. Which of the following antihypertensives would reverse the hypoglycemic effect of antidiabetic pharmacotherapy?

    a. Hydrochlorothiazide (HydroDIURIL)

    b. Timolol (Betimol, others)

    c. Nifedipine (Procardia)

    d. Enalapril (Vasotec)

26. Why must the nurse instruct a patient receiving glipizide (Glucotrol XL) to avoid crushing or chewing the tablets?

    a. The patient may choke.

    b. The effectiveness of the medication would be hindered.

    c. It would cause blood glucose levels to rise too rapidly.

    d. Irritation of the oral mucosa may occur.

27. MAO inhibitors used for treatment of _____ _____ may potentiate hypoglycemic effects when used with _____.

    a. Mood disorders, insulin

    b. Clinical depression, dextrothyroxine

    c. Cushing's syndrome, corticosteroids

    d. Attention deficit/hyperactivity disorder, epinephrine

CALCULATIONS

28. The physician ordered Humulin N U-100 35 units SC, regular Humulin R U-100 20 units. A U-100 insulin syringe is available. What is the total amount of insulin to be given?

29. The physician ordered glipizide 10 mg PO daily. The pharmacy has glipizide 5 mg. How many tablets will the nurse administer?

CASE STUDY APPLICATIONS

30. A 70-year-old male patient has diabetes mellitus type II. The nurse is performing an initial assessment.

    a. In planning this patient's nursing care, which kind of diabetic therapy would he likely require?

    b. Explain the patient teaching needed for this patient, including difficulties that may arise.

31. Over the past 5 years, a 35-year-old firefighter who smokes and is somewhat overweight has begun to develop slightly elevated blood pressure as determined by annual exams. He feels as if he should lose weight and is concerned about his energy level. At his last clinic visit, lab results revealed fasting blood glucose levels at 140 mg/dL. His blood pressure was 150/90 mmHg. The patient was not taking medications for any reported disorder.

    a. What would be expected signs of hyperglycemia in this patient?

    b. In planning this patient's nursing treatment, what preliminary assessments would be needed?

    c. If this patient were to require oral hypoglycemic therapy, on which important teaching areas should the nurse focus?

Adams/Holland, *Student Workbook and Resource Guide for Pharmacology for Nurses* 4th Edition
© 2014 by Pearson Education, Inc.

CHAPTER 45

DRUGS FOR DISORDERS AND CONDITIONS OF THE FEMALE REPRODUCTIVE SYSTEM

FILL IN THE BLANK

From the textbook, find the correct word(s) to complete the statements(s).

1. _____ _____ _____ is the hormone that regulates sperm or egg production; _____ _____ in the female triggers the release of the egg, a process known as ovulation.

2. The permanent cessation of menses, caused by lack of estrogen secretion by the ovaries, is _____.

3. The absence of menstruation is called _____.

4. A class of drugs called _____ is often prescribed for dysfunctional uterine bleeding.

5. The anterior pituitary hormone _____ increases the synthesis of milk within the mammary glands; the posterior pituitary hormone _____ causes milk to be ejected.

Adams/Holland, *Student Workbook and Resource Guide for Pharmacology for Nurses* 4th Edition
© 2014 by Pearson Education, Inc.

MATCHING

For questions 6 through 9, match the drug in column I with its classification in column II.

Column I	Column II
6. _____ norethindrone (Micronor)	a. estrogens
7. _____ terbutaline (Brethine)	b. uterine stimulants
8. _____ mifepristone (Mifeprex) with misoprostol	c. tocolytics
	d. progestin
9. _____ estradiol valerate (Delestrogen)	

For questions 10 through 14, match the drug classification in column I with its indication in column II.

Column I	Column II
10. _____ progestins	a. to prevent conception
11. _____ estrogens	b. for dysfunctional uterine bleeding
12. _____ oral contraceptives	c. for replacement therapy in women and prostate cancer in men
13. _____ oxytocin	d. for premature labor
14. _____ tocolytics	e. to induce labor

MULTIPLE CHOICE

15. The nurse is to administer a triphasic type of oral contraceptive. Which of the following is classified in this manner?

    a. Mircette

    b. Desogen

    c. Ortho-Cyclen

    d. Ortho-Novum

16. Which of the following potential consequences of estrogen loss related to postmenopausal conditions should be included in a teaching plan for the postmenopausal patient?

    a. Insomnia

    b. Sexual disinterest

    c. Mood disturbances

    d. Osteoporosis

17. Which of the following drugs used to treat endometriosis is a GnRH agonist?

    a. Estropipate (Ogen)

    b. Ethinyl estradiol with norethindrone acetate (Activella)

    c. Estradiol (Alora, Climara, Divigel, Elestrin, Estraderm, Estrace, others)

    d. Leuprolide (Eligard, Lupron, Viadur)

18. The nurse understands that which of the following uterine stimulants may also be used for short-term treatment of gastric ulcers?

    a. Oxytocin (Pitocin)

    b. Misoprostol

    c. Dinoprostone (Cervidil, Prepidil, Prostin E$_2$)

    d. Methylergonovine (Methergine)

19. The following medications may be prescribed for the patient with pre-eclampsia. The nurse understands which of these may also be used as an anticonvulsant?

    a. Oxytocin (Pitocin)

    b. Magnesium sulfate

    c. Terbutaline (Brethine)

    d. carboprost (Hemabate)

20. In developing a teaching plan for the patient taking oral contraceptives, the nurse teaches that which of the following may decrease the effectiveness of her chosen method of contraception?

    a. Antibiotics

    b. Antineoplastics

    c. Calcium channel blockers

    d. Antihypertensives

21. Which endocrine gland(s) releases steroid hormones such as estrogen and androgens?

    a. Pituitary gland

    b. Pancreas

    c. Adrenal glands

    d. Hypothalamus

22. The nurse teaches her patient that the oral contraceptive she is taking is effective because it produces a thick cervical mucus. Which of the following medications has this action?

    a. Progesterone (Crinone, Endometrin, Prochieve, Prometrium)

    b. Estradiol (Alora, Climara, Divigel, Elestrin, Estraderm, Estrace, others)

    c. Danazol (Danocrine)

    d. Menotropins (Menopur, Repronex)

23. Which of the following drugs is used for termination of early pregnancy?

    a. Estropipate (Ogen)

    b. Ulipristal (Ella)

    c. Mifepristone (Mifeprex) with misoprostol

    d. Bromocriptine (Parlodel)

24. Which of the following would NOT be included in the teaching plan as a benefit of conjugated estrogen and progestin therapy?

    a. Lowered risk of colon cancer

    b. Reduction in LDL cholesterol

    c. Weight loss

    d. Increase in bone mass

25. The school nurse teaches a group of 9-year-old girls that the function of natural progesterone is which of the following?

    a. To build up the lining of the uterus

    b. To prevent ovulation

    c. To prepare the uterus for implantation of the embryo

    d. To begin the onset of menstrual bleeding

26. The nurse is screening a patient for the appropriateness of oral contraceptive use. The nurse understands that oral contraceptives are contraindicated in patients with which of the following disorders?

    a. Hypertension

    b. Hyperglycemia

    c. Potential for blood clots and stroke

    d. Depression

MAKING CONNECTIONS

27. Relating to women's health care, where would barbiturate thiopental sodium (Pentothal) most likely be used?

    a. Coronary care unit

    b. Sleep disorder clinic

    c. Cancer clinic

    d. Surgical suite

28. What is the classification of interferon alpha-2a?

    a. Alkylating agent

    b. Biologic response modifier

    c. Hormone

    d. Coagulation modifier

29. Which of the following drugs, if given in high doses, could induce hypothyroidism?

    a. Amiodarone (Cordarone)

    b. Finasteride (Proscar)

    c. Repaglinide (Prandin)

    d. Rosiglitazone (Avandia)

30. A diabetic patient is also diagnosed with hypothyroidism. Which of the following reactions to treatment with levothyroxine (Synthroid) would be most expected?

    a. Immediate improvement of symptoms

    b. Initial worsening of symptoms

    c. No change in symptoms

    d. Decreased need for insulin

31. A diabetic patient asks about using stevia as a sugar substitute. Which of the following is NOT true about stevia?

    a. It is an herb found in Paraguay.

    b. It sweetens foods better than sugar.

    c. It is approved by the FDA.

    d. It does not appear to have a negative effect on blood glucose.

CALCULATIONS

32. The physician ordered gonadorelin (Factrel) 100 mcg IVPB added to 100 mL D_5W to be infused over 2 hours. The drop factor is 15 gtt/mL. How many gtt per minute should be given to infuse the total amount in 2 hours?

33. The physician ordered Depo-Provera 100 mg IM. The pharmacy has 400 mg/mL. How many milliliters will the nurse administer?

CASE STUDY APPLICATIONS

34. A 50-year-old female patient is concerned about the unpleasant effects accompanying menopause. Her last menstrual period was several months ago, and she is beginning to experience hot flashes, night sweats, nervousness, and insomnia. The nurse suggests hormone replacement therapy (HRT). The patient states she knows nothing about HRT.

    a. What nursing diagnosis is appropriate for this patient? State the expected outcome for this nursing diagnosis.

    b. State the patient teaching necessary to assist the patient in achieving the expected outcome.

35. A primigravida who is 30 weeks pregnant is in labor. Following rupture of membranes she is receiving oxytocin IV.

    a. What assessment data are necessary for the nurse to gather to monitor for adverse effects?

    b. List nursing actions related to this medication.

CHAPTER 46

DRUGS FOR DISORDERS AND CONDITIONS OF THE MALE REPRODUCTIVE SYSTEM

FILL IN THE BLANK

From the textbook, find the correct word(s) to complete the statements(s).

1. _____ _____ are testosterone-like compounds with hormonal activity.

2. A side effect of testosterone therapy in female patients is the appearance of male sex characteristics or _____.

3. The oral medication first approved for erectile dysfunction in 1998 was _____.

4. _____ _____ _____ is an enlargement of the prostate gland that occurs mostly in men of advanced age.

5. _____ are sex hormones found in male and female patients.

6. Testosterone (Andro) is a category _____ drug and should not be taken if pregnancy is suspected or confirmed.

Adams/Holland, *Student Workbook and Resource Guide for Pharmacology for Nurses* 4th Edition
© 2014 by Pearson Education, Inc.

MATCHING

For questions 7 through 11, match the drug in column I with its classification in column II.

Column I	Column II
7. _____ testosterone	a. androgens
8. _____ doxazosin (Cardura)	b. alpha-adrenergic blocker
9. _____ finasteride (Proscar)	c. alpha-reductase inhibitor
10. _____ danazol	
11. _____ terazosin (Hytrin)	

MULTIPLE CHOICE

12. The patient is concerned about erectile dysfunction. The nurse understands that this condition may be successfully treated with which of the following?

    a. Testosterone (Striant, Androderm, Androgel, Testopel, others)

    b. Sildenafil (Viagra)

    c. Finasteride (Proscar)

    d. doxazosin XL (Cardura XL)

13. When screening for risk factors for erectile dysfunction, the nurse should ask the patient about which of the following diseases?

    a. Diabetes

    b. Hypertension

    c. Benign prostatic hyperplasia (BPH)

    d. Both a and b

14. The nurse must include which of the following adverse effects when providing teaching to a patient receiving anabolic steroids?

    a. Liver damage

    b. Appearance of masculine characteristics

    c. Muscle weakness

    d. Cardiovascular disease

15. The nurse recognizes the patient is taking a natural therapy for BPH when the patient states he is taking which of the following?

    a. Saw palmetto

    b. Ginkgo biloba

    c. St. John's wort

    d. Black cohosh

16. Androgens may be abused by which of the following?

    a. Older adults to improve sexual function

    b. Athletes to improve athletic performance

    c. College students to increase mental acuity

    d. Middle-aged men to arrest hair loss

17. The nurse recognizes which of the following as a symptom of male hypogonadism?

    a. Abundant axillary hair

    b. Decrease in subcutaneous fat

    c. Reduced libido

    d. Hyperactivity

18. The wife of a patient taking anabolic steroids reports to the nurse that her husband has become aggressive. What is the most appropriate response?

    a. "Try speaking to your husband in a low, calm voice."

    b. "Tell me about your behavior prior to his aggressive acts."

    c. "Have you contacted the domestic abuse hotline?"

    d. "This is a common behavioral change related to anabolic steroid use."

19. Instructions for applying a testosterone transdermal patch would include to change sites how frequently?

    a. Every 72 h and rotate sites every 3 days

    b. Every 2 h and rotate sites every 14 days

    c. Every 24 h and rotate sites every 7 days

    d. Every 4 h and rotate sites every 10 days

20. The nurse must routinely monitor which of the following lab values for a patient receiving androgen therapy?

    a. Serum cholesterol

    b. Hematocrit

    c. Prothrombin time

    d. Alpha fetoprotein

21. The nurse understands which of the following drugs to be contraindicated when used concurrently with sildenafil (Viagra)?

    a. Nitroglycerin

    b. Sulfonamides

    c. Sodium bicarbonate

    d. Reglan

22. Which of the following nurses should NOT be assigned to administer medication to the patient receiving finasteride (Proscar)?

    a. Mike, age 29, LPN with male pattern baldness

    b. Lydia, age 35, RN with a cold

    c. Jack, age 40, recently LPN

    d. Susan, age 25, pregnant RN

MAKING CONNECTIONS

23. Stress often has an effect on the release of hormones. Which of the following nervous system components would activate hormonal release at the level of the hypothalamus and adrenal glands?

    a. Somatic nervous system

    b. Sympathetic nervous system

    c. Central nervous system

    d. Sensory nervous system

24. Glucocorticoids would produce an effect at which of the following target receptor locations?

    a. Plasma membrane of the target cell

    b. Cytoplasm of the target cell

    c. Nucleus of the target cell

    d. Cellular component other than the nucleus

25. Cimetidine (Tagamet) is sometimes given to patients who are taking glucocorticoids in order to prevent which disorder?

    a. Hypertension

    b. Constipation

    c. Thromboembolic disease

    d. Peptic ulcer disease

26. The nurse understands an adolescent diabetic's therapeutic regimen is compromised when he states which of the following?

    a. "I'll eat ice cream at the party and take more insulin."

    b. "Taking my blood sugar at the party will be uncomfortable."

    c. "I'll bring my insulin and syringes to the party."

    d. "I can eat party foods that contain protein."

27. In teaching a diabetic patient how to control his blood glucose, the nurse should encourage him to keep the preprandial blood glucose level at which level?

    a. Below 50 mg/dL

    b. Below 110 mg/dL

    c. Above 50 mg/dL

    d. Above 110 mg/dL

CALCULATIONS

28. The physician ordered danazol (Danocrine) 150 mg PO. The pharmacy has 100-mg tablets. How many tablets will the nurse administer?

29. The physician ordered terazosin (Hytrin) 4 mg PO. The pharmacy has 2-mg capsules. How many capsules will the nurse administer?

CASE STUDY APPLICATIONS

30. A 62-year-old male patient is receiving finasteride (Proscar) because of an enlarged prostate. He asks the nurse how he will know if the medication is working and when he can stop taking it.

    a. List the nursing interventions and patient teaching appropriate for this patient.

    b. State specifically how the nurse will evaluate medication effectiveness.

31. A 38-year-old married man has been diagnosed with low testosterone levels. The patient is a type I diabetic and prides himself in his knowledge of herb use related to health.

    a. What assessment data are important for the nurse to obtain before the patient begins androgen therapy?

    b. What nursing interventions and patient education are appropriate for the patient related to his diabetes?

CHAPTER 47

DRUGS FOR BONE AND JOINT DISORDERS

FILL IN THE BLANK

From the textbook, find the correct word(s) to complete the statement(s).

1. _____ _____ _____ is a general term referring to a cluster of disorders that have in common defects in the structure of bone.

2. Calcium levels in the bloodstream are controlled by two endocrine glands, the _____ glands and the _____ gland.

3. Calcium disorders are often associated with _____ _____ disorders.

4. Osteomalacia, referred to as _____ in children, is a disorder characterized by softening of bones without alteration of basic bone structure.

5. Two important disorders characterized by weak and fragile bones are _____ and _____ _____.

6. The hormone responsible for bone resorption is _____ _____; the hormone responsible for bone deposition is _____.

7. Cholecalciferol is converted to an intermediate vitamin form called _____; this intermediate form is transported to the kidneys where enzymes transform it into _____, an active form of vitamin D.

8. The two major forms of calcium used in pharmacotherapy are _____ and _____.

9. Two drug therapies for Paget's disease are _____ and _____.

Adams/Holland, *Student Workbook and Resource Guide for Pharmacology for Nurses* 4th Edition
© 2014 by Pearson Education, Inc.

10. _____ _____ _____ treat rheumatoid arthritis by suppressing autoimmunity.

11. One strategy to prevent hyperuricemia is to use _____, drugs that increase the excretion of uric acid by blocking its reabsorption in the kidney.

MATCHING

For questions 12 through 18, match the drug in column I with its classification in column II.

Column I	Column II
12. _____ calcitriol (Calcijex, Rocaltrol)	a. calcium supplement
13. _____ calcium carbonate (Rolaids, Tums, others)	b. vitamin D therapy
14. _____ allopurinol (Lopurin, Zyloprim)	c. inhibitor of bone resorption
15. _____ etidronate disodium (Didronel)	d. disease-modifying antirheumatic drug
16. _____ azathioprine (Azasan, Imuran)	e. drugs that lower accumulation of uric acid
17. _____ colchicine	
18. _____ alendronate (Fosamax)	

For questions 19 through 23, match the indication in column I with its drug in column II.

Column I	Column II
19. _____ osteomalacia, rickets, and hypocalcemia	a. alendronate sodium (Fosamax)
20. _____ osteoporosis, Paget's disease	b. probenecid (Probalan)
21. _____ gouty arthritis	c. ergocalciferol (Calciferol, Drisdol)
22. _____ rheumatoid arthritis	d. hydroxychloroquine (Plaquenil)
23. _____ osteoarthritis	e. sodium hyaluronate (Hyalgan)

MULTIPLE CHOICE

24. Which of the following statements regarding calcium in the body is NOT true?

    a. When concentrations are too high, sodium permeability decreases across cell membranes.

    b. When concentrations are too low, cell membranes become hyperexcitable.

    c. Calcium must be present for the body to form vitamin D.

    d. Calcium is important for body processes such as blood coagulation and muscle contraction.

25. Diseases and conditions of calcium and vitamin D metabolism include all of the following EXCEPT:

    a. osteomalacia.

    b. rheumatoid arthritis.

    c. osteoporosis.

    d. Paget's disease.

26. Possible etiologies of hypocalcemia include all of the following EXCEPT:

    a. hyposecretion of parathyroid hormone.

    b. digestive-related malabsorption disorders.

    c. lack of adequate intake of calcium-containing foods.

    d. Paget's disease.

27. The nurse is helping an elderly patient with osteoporosis mark her menu. Which of the following choices would be least useful in helping her maintain adequate calcium intake?

    a. Carton of milk for breakfast

    b. Salmon croquette for dinner

    c. Turnip greens for dinner

    d. Baked potato for lunch

28. Calcium gluconate is contraindicated in patients with all of the following conditions EXCEPT:

    a. osteomalacia.

    b. digitalis toxicity.

    c. kidney stones.

    d. cardiac dysrhythmia.

29. Patient teaching regarding vitamin D therapy includes all of the following EXCEPT:

    a. take exactly as directed; it can become toxic if taken in excess quantities.

    b. avoid alcohol and other hepatotoxic drugs.

    c. avoid sunlight exposure due to susceptibility to sunburn.

    d. do not start a low-fat diet unless first discussed with the nurse.

30. All of the following are risk factors for osteoporosis EXCEPT:

    a. anorexia nervosa.

    b. use of estrogen replacement therapy.

    c. high alcohol or caffeine consumption.

    d. advancing age in women.

31. Which statement regarding calcitonin is NOT true?

    a. Obtained from salmon.

    b. Currently available only in oral form.

    c. Increases bone density and reduces the incidence of vertebral fractures.

    d. Indicated for Paget's disease and hypercalcemia.

32. Selective estrogen receptor modulators (SERMs) are contraindicated in patients with all of the following conditions EXCEPT:

    a. thromboembolism.

    b. pregnancy or lactation.

    c. hormone replacement.

    d. postmenopause.

33. Which of the following is NOT a symptom of osteomalacia and/or rickets?

    a. Hypocalcemia

    b. Convulsions

    c. Muscle weakness

    d. Bowlegs and a pigeon breast

34. After analgesic and anti-inflammatory drugs have been tried, which of the following therapies may be used to alter the course of rheumatoid arthritis progression?

    a. Bisphosphonates

    b. Calcitonin therapy

    c. Disease-modifying antirheumatic drugs

    d. Uric acid inhibitors

35. Which of the following gout medications is used for an acute attack and may cause gastric upset?

    a. Colchicine

    b. Allopurinol (Lopurin)

    c. Penicillamine (Cuprimine, Depen)

    d. Sulfasalazine (Azulfidine)

36. Sodium hyaluronate (Hyalgan) is a new therapy for patients with moderate osteoarthritis. Which statement about this drug is NOT true?

    a. It is injected directly into the knee joint.

    b. It coats the articulating cartilage surface.

    c. Patients should avoid strenuous activity for 48 hours after it is administered.

    d. It is used prior to treatments with COX-2 inhibitors and NSAIDs.

37. Which of the following patients is least likely to present with gout?

    a. Pacific Islander

    b. Male

    c. Female

    d. Patient using a thiazide diuretic

MAKING CONNECTIONS

38. Methotrexate can be used to treat rheumatoid arthritis. What other condition is it used for?

    a. Cancer

    b. Pernicious anemia

    c. Cardiac dysrhythmia

    d. Renal failure

39. Promethazine (Phenergan) is a phenothiazine that is used to treat which of the following?

    a. Dysrhythmia

    b. Hypertension

    c. Inflammation

    d. Motion sickness

40. In addition to treating rheumatoid arthritis, hydroxychloroquine (Plaquenil) is also used for which of the following?

    a. Cancer

    b. Pernicious anemia

    c. Malaria

    d. Renal failure

41. Isoniazid can affect serum calcium by causing hypercalcemia. A patient receiving this drug is being treated for which disease?

    a. Peptic ulcers

    b. Tuberculosis infection

    c. Viral infection

    d. Inflammation

42. Diazepam (Valium) is used as an antianxiety agent in many hospitalized patients. What other condition is it used for?

    a. Muscle spasms

    b. Osteomyelitis

    c. Parkinson's disease

    d. Immune disorders

CALCULATIONS

43. The nurse is giving colchicine 0.5-mg tablets for an acute attack of gout. The dose is to be repeated every hour until the patient develops GI symptoms or the pain is relieved. The maximum dose is 4 mg. How many doses can the nurse give before the maximum dose is reached?

44. Hydroxychloroquine (Plaquenil) 400 mg daily is ordered for a patient with rheumatoid arthritis. Available are 200-mg tablets. How many tablets should be given?

CASE STUDY APPLICATIONS

45. A 74-year-old male patient with primary gout has just started taking allopurinol (Lopurin), 100 mg daily. He is reporting symptoms of gastric upset and intermittent episodes of extreme pain in the joints.

    a. What education should the nurse provide regarding these symptoms and their treatment?

    b. What education should the nurse provide regarding possible adverse effects?

    c. What laboratory tests should the nurse monitor to determine the longer term effects of allopurinol?

46. A 28-year-old type I diabetic with renal failure is on hemodialysis. The nurse brings her a.m. medications that include Rocaltrol and calcium tablets.

    a. The patient asks the nurse why she is receiving vitamin D and calcium, because she does not have a bone disease and is too young for osteoporosis. How does the nurse explain this to her?

    b. What patient teaching regarding vitamin D therapy would the nurse give this patient?

    c. What information regarding calcium supplements should the nurse give her?

47. A 78-year-old female patient has been admitted to the hospital with a vertebral compression fracture. Now that her pain has been controlled, she is asking the nurse questions about prevention of further problems of this nature.

    a. The patient wants to know what causes the bones to come brittle in elderly people. What explanation will the nurse give her?

    b. What drug therapy is likely to be prescribed to treat this patient's osteoporosis?

    c. What education will this patient need regarding the use of her prescriptions for Fosamax and Evista?

CHAPTER 48

DRUGS FOR SKIN DISORDERS

FILL IN THE BLANK

From the textbook, find the correct word(s) to complete the statement(s).

1. Drugs used to promote the shedding of old skin are called _____ agents.

2. Mites cause a skin disorder called _____.

3. Vitamin A–like compounds providing resistance to bacterial infection by reducing oil production and the occurrence of clogged pores are called _____.

4. _____ are oral or topical agents that produce a photosensitive reaction when exposed to UV light, as in the case of psoriasis treatment.

5. Itching associated with dry, scaly skin is called _____.

6. Other than keratolytic agents, two classes of drugs offer some protection against acne, including _____ and _____ _____.

7. A skin disorder with symptoms resembling an allergic reaction is called atopic dermatitis or _____.

Adams/Holland, *Student Workbook and Resource Guide for Pharmacology for Nurses* 4th Edition
© 2014 by Pearson Education, Inc.

MATCHING

For questions 8 through 14, match the drug in column I with its classification in column II.

Column I

8. _____ benzoyl peroxide (Clearasil, Fostex, others)

9. _____ fluticasone propionate, cream (Cutivate)

10. _____ etanercept (Enbrel)

11. _____ azelaic acid (Azelex, Finacea)

12. _____ permethrin (Elimite)

13. _____ benzocaine (Solarcaine)

14. _____ sulfacetamide sodium (Cetamide, Klaron, others)

Column II

a. scabicide/pediculicide

b. sunburn/minor irritation agent

c. acne and acne-related agent

d. topical glucocorticoid

e. psoriatic agent

For questions 15 through 19, match the symptom in column I with its description in column II.

Column I

15. _____ erythema

16. _____ pruritus

17. _____ sunburn

18. _____ open comedones

19. _____ closed comedones

Column II

a. blackheads

b. whiteheads

c. intense itching

d. redness

e. "first-degree" injury

MULTIPLE CHOICE

20. Drugs to treat oily skin would most likely be used for which of the following disorders?

    a. Atopic dermatitis

    b. Contact dermatitis

    c. Seborrheic dermatitis

    d. Stasis dermatitis

21. Which of the following medications decreases comedone formation and increases extrusion of comedones from the skin?

    a. Benzoyl peroxide (Clearasil, Fostex, others)

    b. Tretinoin (Avita, Retin-A, others)

    c. Calcipotriene (Dovonex)

    d. Hydrocortisone

22. Which of the following medications is administered topically for psoriasis?

    a. Calcipotriene (Dovonex)

    b. Acitretin (Soriatane)

    c. Etanercept (Enbrel)

    d. Methotrexate (Rheumatrex, Trexall)

23. Which of the following medications would NOT be useful for minor insect bites?

    a. Benzocaine (Solarcaine)

    b. Dibucaine (Nupercainal)

    c. Tetracaine (Pontocaine)

    d. Salicylic acid (Salex, Neutrogena, others)

24. Which of the following treatments would NOT be used to promote the shedding of old skin?

    a. UVA/UVB

    b. Methoxsalen

    c. Coal tar (Balnetar, Cutar, others)

    d. Benzoyl peroxide (Clearasil, Fostex, others)

25. Which of the following statements about benzocaine is true?

    a. When applied to the ear, mouth, or throat, it produces minor irritation.

    b. It is more appropriate for sunburn than for pruritus or insect bites.

    c. Drug sensitivity is rare.

    d. It should not be applied to an open wound.

26. Which of the following is an OTC medication for acne?

    a. Clindamycin and tretinoin (Veltin, Ziana)

    b. Tazarotene (Avage, Tazorac)

    c. Benzoyl peroxide with erythromycin (Benzamycin)

    d. Metronidazole (MetroCream, MetroGel)

27. Exposure to perfume, cosmetics, detergents, or latex is associated with which of the following disorders?

    a. Atopic dermatitis

    b. Contact dermatitis

    c. Seborrheic dermatitis

    d. Stasis dermatitis

28. Topical glucocorticoids are a common treatment for all of the following EXCEPT:

    a. psoriasis.

    b. rosacea.

    c. pruritus.

    d. dermatitis.

29. Which of the following is contraindicated in conjunction with phototherapy for the treatment of psoriasis?

    a. Tar and anthralin

    b. Keratolytic pastes

    c. Psoralens

    d. Cyclosporine

30. This drug is an alternative scabicide to lindane (Kwell) available by prescription as a 10% cream.

    a. Crotamiton (Eurax)

    b. Permethrin (Nix)

    c. Malathion (Ovide)

    d. Bacitracin ointment

31. Use of isotretinoin (Accutane) is contraindicated in patients with all of these conditions EXCEPT:

    a. acne vulgaris.

    b. severe depression and suicidal tendencies.

    c. seizures treated with carbamazepine.

    d. diabetes treated with oral agents.

32. Which vitamin is synthesized by the skin?

    a. Vitamin A

    b. Vitamin D

    c. Vitamin E

    d. Vitamin K

MAKING CONNECTIONS

33. Methotrexate may be used to treat psoriasis. Which other conditions is it used for?

    a. Gout and rheumatoid arthritis

    b. Rheumatoid arthritis and certain cancers

    c. Systemic fungal infections and certain cancers

    d. Urinary tract infections and peptic ulcers

34. Topical metronidazole (MetroCream, MetroGel) is used to treat rosacea. Extensive used would treat which of the following?

    a. To decrease glucose levels in the blood

    b. To decrease lipid levels in the blood

    c. To treat inflammatory papules

    d. To treat skin sensitivity

35. What drug is used as a local anesthetic and an antidysrhythmic?

    a. Warfarin (Coumadin)

    b. Propranolol (Inderal)

    c. Infliximab (Remicade)

    d. Lidocaine (Xylocaine)

36. Which is among the first-line drugs used for allergic rhinitis?

    a. NSAIDs

    b. Sympathomimetics

    c. Glucocorticoids

    d. Cytokines

CASE STUDY APPLICATIONS

37. A 9-year-old female child is brought to the pediatrician by her mother for an immunization. As the nurse gives the injection, the nurse notices that the child has nits clinging to her hair. A quick assessment shows that the child appears to be clean and well cared for. When the nurse points out the problem to her mother, she confesses that she has used an OTC treatment for the lice, which her daughter got at a friend's sleepover. She is obviously uncomfortable and blurts out, "We're not like that—we are clean people."

    a. What teaching must the nurse do regarding the use of lindane?

    b. Whom must the mother notify of her daughter's pediculosis?

    c. What information can the nurse give the mother and daughter to prevent this problem from recurring?

38. The nurse is working at a walk-in clinic in Florida. A 20-year-old college student visiting from Minnesota on spring break presents with complaints of severe sunburn.

    a. What other assessments would the nurse need?

    b. What interventions might help the pain and other symptoms of sunburn?

    c. Promotion of wellness is one goal in the care plan. What information should be given to the young man regarding prevention and sequelae of sunburn?

39. A 17-year-old male stops by the school nurse's office to "hang out." After some preliminary conversation, he confides to the nurse that he is worried about his complexion, and that nothing he has tried has cleared up his severe acne. He is afraid he will be "scarred for life" and asks if there are any other medications to help him. He also wants to know why he has such a bad case of acne, and his friend has hardly any.

    a. What can the nurse tell the patient about the causes of acne?

    b. What assessments must be made prior to starting Accutane?

    c. What other information should be assessed regarding the patient's lifestyle and hygiene habits?

Adams/Holland, *Student Workbook and Resource Guide for Pharmacology for Nurses* 4th Edition
© 2014 by Pearson Education, Inc.

CHAPTER 49

DRUGS FOR EYE
AND EAR DISORDERS

FILL IN THE BLANK

From the textbook, find the correct word(s) to complete the statement(s).

1. In patients who have glaucoma, increased intraocular pressure is caused by a _____ in the _____ of aqueous humor or _____ _____ of aqueous humor.

2. A type of slower developing glaucoma where the iris does not cover the trabecular meshwork is referred to as _____ _____.

3. Drugs that cause the pupils to constrict are called _____.

4. Drugs that cause the pupils to dilate are referred to as _____.

5. Drugs that cause relaxation of ciliary muscles are called _____.

6. Swimmer's ear is sometimes referred to as _____ _____.

7. Inflammation of the middle ear is called _____ _____.

8. Inflammation of the mastoid sinus is called _____.

Adams/Holland, *Student Workbook and Resource Guide for Pharmacology for Nurses* 4th Edition
© 2014 by Pearson Education, Inc.

MATCHING

For questions 9 through 14, match the drug in column I with its action in column II.

	Column I	Column II
9.	_____ pilocarpine (Isopto Carpine, Pilopine)	a. increase the outflow of aqueous humor
10.	_____ timolol (Betimol, Timoptic, others)	b. decrease the formation of aqueous humor
11.	_____ dorzolamide (Trusopt)	
12.	_____ brinzolamide (Azopt)	
13.	_____ dipivefrin HCl (Propine)	
14.	_____ latanoprost (Xalatan)	

For questions 15 through 22, match the antiglaucoma drug in column I with its classification in column II.

	Column I	Column II
15.	_____ pilocarpine (Isopto Carpine, Pilopine)	a. miotic, direct-acting cholinergic agonist
16.	_____ methazolamide (Neptazane)	b. sympathomimetic
17.	_____ isosorbide (Ismotic)	c. prostaglandin analog
18.	_____ dipivefrin HCl (Propine)	d. beta blocker
19.	_____ carteolol (Ocupress)	e. alpha$_2$-adrenergic agonist, direct acting
20.	_____ travaprost (Travatan)	f. carbonic anhydrase inhibitor
21.	_____ betaxolol (Betoptic)	g. osmotic diuretic
22.	_____ apraclonidine (Iopidine)	

MULTIPLE CHOICE

23. Which of the following types of medications may contribute to the development of glaucoma?

    a. Beta blockers

    b. Corticosteroids

    c. Antibiotics

    d. Calcium channel blockers

24. Which of the following best describes closed-angle glaucoma?

    a. Is referred to as chronic, simple glaucoma

    b. Develops when the iris is pushed over the area where the aqueous fluid normally drains

    c. Develops more slowly than open-angle glaucoma

    d. Is best treated by drugs that decrease the formation of aqueous humor

25. Which of the following classes of drugs for eye procedures should NOT be used for patients with glaucoma?

    a. Mydriatic (sympathomimetic) drugs

    b. Cycloplegic (anticholinergic) drugs

    c. Osmotic diuretics

    d. Carbonic anhydrase inhibitors

26. When used for glaucoma, one drawback of prostaglandin analogs is that they do which of the following?

    a. Change pigmentation of the eye

    b. Reduce blood pressure

    c. Increase urine output

    d. Block sympathetic impulses

27. Which of the following medications is converted to epinephrine in the eye?

    a. Tafluprost (Zioptan)

    b. Carbachol (Miostat)

    c. Dipivefrin HCl (Propine)

    d. Echothiophate iodide (Phospholine iodide)

28. Which class of drugs used for eye examinations has the potential to produce unfavorable CNS effects?

    a. Osmotic diuretics

    b. Sympathomimetic drugs

    c. Anticholinergic drugs

    d. Cholinergic agonists

29. Major risk factors associated with glaucoma include all of the following EXCEPT:

    a. hypertension.

    b. migraine headaches.

    c. ethnic origin.

    d. epilepsy.

30. Which of the following statements regarding closed-angle (acute) glaucoma is NOT true?

    a. It is usually unilateral.

    b. The iris is pushed over the area where the fluid normally drains.

    c. It is frequently seen in persons of Caucasian race.

    d. It constitutes an emergency situation.

31. Which of the following statements regarding beta-blocking agents is NOT true?

    a. They are contraindicated in persons who are allergic to sulfa.

    b. Before the discovery of prostaglandin analogs, they were the preferred drugs for glaucoma therapy.

    c. They generally produce fewer ocular adverse effects than other autonomic drugs.

    d. They may produce systemic side effects such as bronchoconstriction, bradycardia, and hypotension.

32. In which patient would the use of carbonic anhydrase inhibitors be contraindicated?

    a. A patient with asthma-producing bronchospasms

    b. A patient with an allergy to sulfonamides

    c. A patient with open-angle glaucoma

    d. A patient with a history of third-degree AV block

33. The nurse is teaching an elderly patient to instill her own eye drops. How will the nurse explain the procedure?

    a. "Tilt the head back and toward the side of the affected eye."

    b. "Tilt the head back and toward the side of the unaffected eye."

    c. "Instill the drops to the center of the cornea, blink, and wipe the eye."

    d. "Lift the upper lid by the lashes, and drop the medication into the sac."

34. When teaching a family member to instill eye drops for an elderly patient, the nurse will include all of the following EXCEPT:

    a. Apply gentle pressure for 30 seconds to the inner canthus after instilling.

    b. Wait 5 minutes before instilling another type of drops.

    c. There is no need to remove the patient's contact lenses.

    d. Eye medication should be refrigerated.

35. What is the basic course of treatment for ear infection?

    a. Antibiotics

    b. Corticosteroids

    c. Earwax removal agents

    d. Irrigation with a bulb syringe

36. Which of the following regarding ciprofloxacin (Cipro otic) ear drops is true?

    a. It is used primarily in cases of ruptured eardrum.

    b. It is indicated to relieve pain and reduce fever.

    c. It is a commonly used topical antibiotic.

    d. It is used primarily to treat otitis media.

37. When instilling ear drops, all of the following are correct EXCEPT:

    a. run warm water over the bottle to warm the drops.

    b. the procedure generally involves gentle lavage of the wax-impacted ear with tepid water using an asepto syringe.

    c. the patient should lie on the side opposite the affected ear for 5 minutes after instillation.

    d. the area should not be massaged to prevent systemic drug effects.

MAKING CONNECTIONS

38. Cholinergic agonists exert an effect in the body through which type of receptor?

    a. Nicotinic

    b. Muscarinic

    c. Dopaminergic

    d. Serotonergic

39. Beta blockers are examples of which class of antidysrhythmic drugs?

    a. Class I

    b. Class II

    c. Class III

    d. Class IV

40. What is one important respiratory effect of beta blockers?

    a. Bronchospasm

    b. Bronchodilation

    c. Increased release of surfactant

    d. Hyperventilation

41. What is the most serious adverse effect of taking potassium-sparing diuretics and salt substitutes at the same time?

    a. Hyperkalemia

    b. Hypokalemia

    c. Edema

    d. Dehydration

42. In addition to glaucoma, the carbonic anhydrase inhibitor drug group is also prescribed for which of the following?

    a. Seizures

    b. Coagulation disorders

    c. Psoriasis

    d. Malaria

CALCULATIONS

43. The patient has an order for acetazolamide (Diamox) 250 mg PO tid. What is the total amount of Diamox the patient will receive in 24 hours?

44. The patient has acute glaucoma. Pilocarpine HCl (Isopto Carpine) has been ordered 1 drop every 5 minutes for 6 doses. Would the nurse question this order? Why or why not?

CASE STUDY APPLICATIONS

45. A male patient was recently diagnosed with open-angle glaucoma. Intraocular pressure is currently being controlled with miotic medications, including latanoprost (Xalatan). The patient wants to know if there is a permanent cure and if continued treatment will be necessary.

    a. The nurse's care plan includes interventions related to patient education. What patient teaching must the nurse do for this patient regarding his disease?

    b. One of this patient's nursing diagnoses reads "*Deficient Knowledge* related to therapeutic regimen as evidenced by patient's inability to tell indications and side effects of antiglaucoma medications." What specific information regarding the use of latanoprost (Xalatan) must the nurse give this patient?

    c. List some general nursing interventions that would be important for a patient with glaucoma.

    d. How would the nurse evaluate the effectiveness of this patient's glaucoma medications?

46. A 5-year-old boy is brought to the pediatrician's office by his mother who states he has been crying, running a temperature of 102°F, and complaining of an earache. The nurse's assessment reveals bulging, reddened eardrums, and bloody drainage in the left ear. The mother states that she has been using chewable baby aspirin for his fever, and that she has another child at home using "ear drops, and he hates those cold things going into his ears." A diagnosis of otitis media is made by the pediatrician, and an oral antibiotic is prescribed.

    a. What other assessments must the nurse make regarding the use of antibiotics by this patient?

    b. The patient's mother obviously has a lack of knowledge about her son's medications and treatments. What interventions could the nurse include in the care plan to address this patient problem?

47. A female patient has come to the clinic with complaints of mild hearing loss and a sensation of fullness with intermittent ringing of the ears. Upon assessment with the otoscope, the nurse observes a dark mass in the ear canal.

    a. What other assessments should be made prior to treating this problem?

    b. How would the problem be treated?

ANSWER KEY

Chapter 1

1. John Jacob Abel
2. chemists, natural products
3. synthesize
4. quality of life
5. medicines
6. disease
7. prevention, suffering
8. biologic
9. Over-the-counter

10. b	11. c	12. a	13. d	14. b	15. a
16. d	17. c	18. c	19. d	20. d	21. c
22. d	23. b	24. c	25. d	26. d	27. a

28. a. It is important to cover the following points in a teaching plan for a patient with mild constipation:
    - Natural alternatives usually cost less than OTC drugs.
    - Natural alternatives tend to produce fewer side effects.
    - Mild constipation can also be treated with diet changes: Try using high-fiber products and increasing water consumption.
    - If constipation persists, the patient needs to make an appointment for assessment with a nurse.

    b. A nursing history would include the patient's medical history including bowel health, nutritional history, and medication history. It is important to evaluate what OTC medications have been taken in the past and what prescription drugs are being taken. Remember to assess both current and past herbal and alternative therapies. Also assess social history, which includes use of alcohol, tobacco, and street drugs.

29. a. A patient can have a drug reaction to OTC, generic, or trade-name medications. The important nursing action is to assess what reaction the patient is having and how life threatening it is for her. Life-threatening reactions include those that affect the heart and lungs. If the patient is having difficulty breathing or is having a blood pressure or heart abnormality, then she needs to seek emergency care. All drug reactions should be taken seriously. A nurse should be consulted for all drug reactions.

    b. It is important for the patient to know that all prescription drugs are thoroughly tested because of the Food, Drug and Cosmetic Act of 1938. The Food and Drug Administration (FDA) must approve a drug before it is sold in the United States. The FDA also oversees administration of herbal products and dietary supplements. The Federal Trade Commission ensures that the advertising of OTC medications and health food supplements is not fraudulent, deceptive, or unsubstantiated.

Chapter 2

1. therapeutic
2. pharmacologic
3. prototype
4. chemical, generic, trade
5. chemical
6. combination drugs
7. bioavailability
8. pharmacoeconomics

9. b	10. a	11. d	12. c	13. a	14. c
15. d	16. a	17. b	18. a	19. a	20. d
21. c					

22. a. Generic and trade products have identical doses; however, the ingredients in the generic product may be slightly different. In many states, the pharmacist is allowed to dispense generic equivalents unless the patient or nurse specifies that a trade product is required. In Florida, if a drug is on the negative drug formulary list, it must be dispensed in its trade form only. It is best that the nurse check the state requirements for dispensing of trade versus generic products.

    b. Tylenol is an analgesic nonnarcotic. It is not a controlled substance. In the United States, controlled substances are drugs whose use is restricted by the Controlled Substances Act of 1970.

Chapter 3

1. enteral
2. topical
3. five rights

263

Adams/Holland, *Student Workbook and Resource Guide for Pharmacology for Nurses* 4th Edition
© 2014 by Pearson Education, Inc.

4. oral

5. Sublingual

6. Suppositories, enemas

7. oral

8. intramuscular

9. transdermal

10. Inhalations, instillations, irrigations

11. a   12. b   13. b   14. a   15. c   16. b
17. c   18. a   19. b   20. c   21. b   22. d
23. d   24. c   25. d   26. a   27. b   28. b
29. b   30. c   31. d   32. b   33. d   34. c

35. a. The nurse must take a detailed personal, family, and sexual health history when assisting the patient in a choice of contraception.

b. Oral contraceptive agents are effective and convenient; however, missing a daily dose means risking pregnancy. Therefore, for an active lifestyle, this may not be the most desirable approach. On the other hand, an oral medication may be less bothersome than injections, patches, or vaginal inserts. Injections or implants may last a long time, but they may be initially painful or subject to infection. In addition, these approaches may be uncomfortable, as may vaginal inserts. Vaginal inserts might be used less routinely because they are sometimes messy, inconvenient, and less reliable. The nurse should help the patient weigh every disadvantage against the convenience of taking medication less frequently.

36. a. Because the patient is nauseated and has diarrhea, oral medications or suppositories would probably not be recommended unless the nausea and diarrhea were not severe enough to interfere with the drug therapy. Because the source of discomfort is the gastrointestinal tract, topical drugs would most likely do little good to relieve discomfort; also, in elderly patients, the skin is usually sensitive. Alternatives might be drugs administered by the parenteral route, for example, in an intramuscular or subcutaneous injection.

b. Effectiveness of the route of medication can be evaluated by collecting data about the resolution of presenting symptoms.

Chapter 4

1. absorption, distribution, metabolism, excretion

2. blood–brain, fetal–placental

3. Metabolism

4. first-pass effect

5. Absorption

6. dissolution

7. excretion

8. Toxic concentration

9. therapeutic range

10. loading

11. a   12. b   13. a   14. b   15. a   16. b
17. c   18. b   19. c   20. a   21. a   22. c
23. d   24. a

25. a. Because the patient is obese, the medications may be dissolved in the fat and accumulate there, and then slowly be released. Hypertension and diabetes can alter drug distribution as these disorders are associated with compromised renal function. When renal function is compromised, drug dosing must be reduced to account for changes in metabolic and excretion function.

b. The patient's anxiety should be reduced. Half-life of the drug should be considered by the nurse. If the patient is experiencing side effects of the antianxiety drugs, then the nurse should consider renal and hepatic function as a potential problem, increasing the plasma half-life.

c. The primary site of excretion for all medications is the kidney. The nurse should be checking intake and output on this patient.

26. a. This patient has been abusing alcohol, which will affect hepatic function. He is 60 years old and therefore has some degree of vessel narrowing.

b. Because of the history of alcohol abuse and the age of the patient, medication dosing may be reduced to lessen the chance of toxicity.

c. The nurse should assess the renal system. If renal blood flow has been impaired, then excretion of medications will be slow and side or toxic effects may be seen in the postprocedure period.

Chapter 5

1. Pharmacodynamics

2. receptor

3. Potency, efficacy

4. frequency distribution

5. 50

6. lethal

7. therapeutic index

8. lower

9. graded dose-response

10. Antagonists

11. b   12. a   13. b   14. a   15. a   16. b
17. a   18. a   19. a   20. c   21. d   22. b
23. c   24. c   25. d

26. a. Determine the age of the patient. Identify how often the analgesic is used for pain relief and how efficacious the medication has been. Identify if the dosage is standard and safe. Evaluate the therapeutic index for this drug.

b. *Chronic Pain* (©2012 NANDA-I) related to history of migraine headaches

c. Has there been enough time for the medication to be absorbed and distributed? Does the patient need a more potent drug? Is the agonist/antagonist formulation of this drug not appropriate for this patient? Are drug–drug interactions occurring? Are drug–food interactions occurring?

27. a. What antibiotics are the patients taking? Are the doses standard, safe, and potent? Have the patients taken the drugs long enough to consider the slow results unreasonable? Is this an efficacy issue?

b. The patient exhibits the following signs of wound healing: well-approximated wound edges, no drainage 48 hours after wound is closed, and no inflammatory response past day 5 after the injury.

c. Wound edges opening, drainage, inflammation, pain, fever

Chapter 6

1. nursing diagnoses
2. evaluation
3. observation
4. nursing process

5. f	6. e	7. d	8. c	9. g	10. h
11. a	12. c	13. d	14. b	15. a	16. b
17. a	18. d	19. b	20. a	21. c	22. d
23. c	24. a	25. a	26. b	27. b	28. c
29. a					

30. a. This adolescent patient has a risk for noncompliance for treatment of a condition with potentially long-term adverse effects to major organs of the body.

b. *Noncompliance to Treatment* (©2012 NANDA-I) related to failure to follow treatment regimen as evidenced by blood glucose levels of over 400

31. a. The priority intervention is to establish the need for and use of an interpreter to communicate with the patient. This will enable the nurse to communicate an effective plan of care to the patient and reduce the risk for legal implications.

b. Language, culture, lifestyle, education, low income, health care beliefs

32. a. The potential exists for withdrawal adverse effects from the abused drugs and the potential to require additional medication for pain relief. Also, there is a potential for noncompliance to treatment related to drug dependency.

b. The patient will follow established plan of care as an inpatient and outpatient. The patient will enroll in a substance abuse recovery program and be in compliance with goals of the program. The desired outcome will be for a complete recovery from the trauma and substance abuse.

Chapter 7

1. preventable, patient harm
2. sentinel events
3. medication reconciliation

4. clarified (or verified), administered
5. warfarin (Coumadin)

6. b	7. d	8. a	9. c	10. b	11. d
12. d	13. c	14. a	15. b	16. d	17. d
18. a	19. b	20. c	21. c	22. c	23. c
24. d	25. d	26. a	27. a	28. d	29. c
30. b					

31. a. Assessment is the first step of the nursing process. Subjective data (complaining of a headache) and objective data (vital signs) are both used.

b. The nurse should have explored reasons why the patient stopped the medication. Once the reason is determined the nurse could discuss substituting a different drug as an alternative pain therapy with the health care provider.

32. a. *Risk for Injury* (©2012 NANDA-I) related to excessive anticoagulation as evidenced by increased dosage of anticoagulant medication

b. Implementation would include monitoring the patient for signs and symptoms of increased clotting time and elevated prothrombin time.

33. a. The nurse needs to find out when the patient took her last dose of lithium, her prescribed dose, and her current lithium level. When a patient is experiencing a period of sodium depletion (e.g., use of diuretics, dehydration), the proximal tubule of the kidney will reabsorb sodium and lithium in an effort to prevent the depletion of these salts. Consequently, lithium serum levels rise and may lead to lithium toxicity. Finding out the serum lithium level would provide important information about possible toxicity. Therapeutic levels of lithium are 0.5 to 1.2 mEq/L. Toxic levels are most serious when serum lithium levels exceed 2 mEq/L.

b. Yes. If the patient's lithium level is elevated, administering another dose of lithium would increase the symptoms of toxicity. Nurses should always review recent laboratory data and other information in the patient's chart before administering medications, especially those drugs, such as lithium, that have a narrow margin of safety.

c. The nurse should question the order. If the nurse administers the dose and the patient develops more serious symptoms, most likely both the nurse and the health care provider are liable. The standard by which the nurse is judged is whether the actions were what a reasonable and prudent nurse would have done when faced with a similar dilemma.

d. *Deficient Fluid Volume.* (©2012 NANDA-I) The patient will verbalize an understanding of sodium and fluid requirements when taking lithium. *Risk for Poisoning* (©2012 NANDA-I) related to lithium toxicity. The patient will maintain a therapeutic serum level by regular monitoring of blood lithium levels.

e. Teaching would include information about changing sodium intake, taking new medications, and other changes that may cause lithium toxicity or increased excretion of lithium.

34. a. Although this is clearly an astute judgment and is a deviation from the precise order, most nurses would not consider this a medication error. No harm has occurred. Nurses who practice in clinical agencies need to understand and follow policies and procedures governing medication administration for the organization in which they practice. These policies and procedures establish the standards of care for that particular hospital or organization, and it is important that nurses adhere to those established policies and procedures. Common errors relate to failing to administer a medication at the prescribed time. For example, an agency policy may identify that it is permissible to give a medication 30 minutes early or 30 minutes late for medications taken four times a day. The standards of care and the agency's policy manual are designed to help the nurse reduce medication errors and maintain patient safety.

    b. To make allowances without consulting the prescribing care provider is not wise. It would be better for the nurse to consult with the provider and have the order changed. The nurse should also indicate on the medication administration record that the medication was given at 8 a.m. and omitted at 10 a.m.

Chapter 8

1. growth
2. development
3. holistic
4. preimplantation, embryonic, fetal
5. maternal kidney, excretion
6. decreases, lower
7. teratogen
8. polypharmacy

9. a	10. e	11. b	12. c	13. d	14. b
15. b	16. a	17. a	18. c	19. d	20. c
21. b	22. c	23. d	24. b	25. a	26. c
27. c	28. c	29. c	30. c	31. a	32. a

33. a. The skeleton and other major organ systems are developed by week 8. Because substance abuse acts as a teratogen, all or some of the major organs could be affected.

    b. The woman may deliver a neonate that has multiple developmental anomalies.

    c. Drugs and other chemicals ingested by the mother may cross the placental barrier and affect the developing fetus.

34. a. Middle-age adults are sometimes called the "sandwich generation" because they are caring for children, grandchildren, and aging parents.

    b. They must opt for lifestyle changes such as limiting lipid intake, maintaining optimum weight, and exercising to improve overall health.

    c. Cardiovascular disease, hypertension, obesity, arthritis, cancer, and anxiety

35. a. Polypharmacy

    b. The chances for drug interactions and adverse reactions dramatically increase.

    c. Although the nurse should avoid preconceived ideas that all older adults are physically and cognitively impaired, a careful assessment of hearing, vision, and mental status is necessary.

Chapter 9

1. holistic
2. perceptions, preferred modes
3. cultural competence
4. lack of access
5. pharmacogenetics

6. c	7. e	8. f	9. b	10. a	11. c
12. d	13. d	14. b	15. b	16. a	17. b
18. c	19. d	20. a	21. b	22. a	23. a
24. b	25. d				

26. a. Assess the patient's cultural background, level of income, lifestyle, religious beliefs, use of nonprescription drugs, and whether there are other environmental factors (such as the husband's alcoholic parents living with her) that may contribute to her child's future alcohol abuse or influence her well-being. This patient should also be assessed for the possibility of domestic violence.

    b. Alcoholism has both social and biologic components. Some persons are more sensitive to alcohol based on their genetic makeup. Alcoholism may develop in people who are exposed to socially accepted drinking. It may be influenced by culture, environment, poverty, and traumatic experiences.

    c. Referrals for this patient may include a community group such as Al-Anon or her church. She also needs to enlist the support of her nonalcoholic family. She may need referrals for WIC or other financial assistance. (If the assessment for domestic violence is positive, appropriate referrals should be made.)

27. a. Adverse effects of the antihypertensives should be assessed—especially whether they are causing impotence. Also, the patient's knowledge of the use of the medications and how to take them should be evaluated.

    b. He should be instructed in the correct dosage schedule and side effects that may occur. The patient needs to know that abruptly discontinuing antihypertensives has been known to cause strokes.

28. a. Other types of pain-relieving measures that may be acceptable to this patient include guided imagery, biofeedback, acupuncture, therapeutic massage, heat, cold, and TENS unit usage.

    b. Find out the patient's religion and offer her the option of a consultation with a minister regarding the use of stronger medications. Find out what she has done in the past to relieve her pain, and do this, if possible.

c. Possibly a nonnarcotic pain reliever would give some relief. Acetaminophen, aspirin, and ibuprofen do not cause the drowsiness often associated with narcotics.

Chapter 10

1. healing power
2. reduce, medications
3. judgmental
4. woody tissue, stems, or bark
5. active chemicals
6. Dietary Supplement Health and Education (DSHEA)
7. e   8. d   9. d   10. a   11. b   12. b
13. b   14. d   15. e   16. c   17. d   18. c
19. a   20. c   21. d   22. d   23. c   24. b
25. c   26. b   27. a   28. d   29. c   30. a
31. d   32. d   33. a   34. b
35. a. The nurse should find out what herbs the patient is planning on using, and determine whether he is aware of possible side effects and herb–drug interactions.

b. Many herbal supplements cause increased effects from warfarin and digoxin. The patient should be informed that he may experience increased tendency to bleed and possibly digitalis toxicity. Herbal preparations should not be taken without consulting his health care provider. Since the patient may take the herbals in spite of the nurse's warning, he should be instructed in signs and symptoms to report. Symptoms of bleeding include bruises, bleeding gums, and hematuria. Digoxin toxicity symptoms include anorexia, nausea, and yellow haloes around objects.

c. Some patients may be allergic to one of the many chemicals in herbals. Patients should start by using the smallest amount possible until it is determined whether they have an allergy to any component of the substance.

36. a. The patient may be experiencing serotonin syndrome caused by the combination of the Prozac and the St. John's wort.

b. Combining St. John's wort with tricyclic antidepressants such as Elavil or Tofranil may cause serotonin syndrome. MAOIs in combination with St. John's wort may cause hypertensive crisis.

37. a. The nurse should monitor liver function studies (AST, ALT) because the combination of echinacea and methotrexate may result in hepatotoxicity.

b. Because this patient is already combining a prescription drug with an herbal that is known to have an adverse interaction, the possibility of herb–drug interactions should be stressed. The patient should also be taught that herbal supplements are not FDA tested

and may not do what they claim to do. He should be made aware of the possibility of an allergic reaction to an ingredient in the preparation.

c. This goal is probably not realistic, as the patient is already using an herbal preparation, although he is not happy with the results at the present time. The nurse should attempt to understand what the patient is trying to accomplish by using the herbal preparation and be prepared to offer him alternatives to meet his needs. He may need a new prescription, or possibly wish to combine herbals with prescription medications. Open communication and a nonjudgmental attitude on the part of the nurse will encourage the patient to explore possibilities and decide upon what is best for his situation. A more realistic goal might be to have the patient verbalize possible herb–drug interactions related to the echinacea prior to discharge.

Chapter 11

1. alcohol, nicotine
2. opium, marijuana, cocaine
3. tolerance, cross-tolerance
4. physical dependence, psychological dependence
5. Addiction
6. crack cocaine
7. benzodiazepine
8. methadone, buprenorphine, naloxone
9. tolerance
10. withdrawal syndrome
11. a   12. b   13. c   14. d   15. b   16. b
17. d   18. a   19. d   20. e   21. a   22. b
23. c   24. a   25. a   26. a   27. b   28. b
29. c   30. a   31. d   32. d   33. c   34. d
35. a   36. d   37. b
38. a. Marijuana can damage the lungs and increase the chance for cancer of the lung.

b. Marijuana causes psychological dependence. It is also considered the "gateway" drug: It opens the patient to opportunities for poor judgment and the possibility of taking other drugs when the person is "high" on marijuana.

c. Lung cancer is a risk in those people who smoke marijuana.

39. a. There is substantial evidence to suggest that genetics plays a major role in addiction. However, many factors could increase the likelihood of someone abusing alcohol, as well as other addictive drugs. If a person has a genetic predisposition to substance abuse, it is best to carefully weigh the risks of addiction before consuming alcohol or other addicting substances.

b. When did the patient last consume alcohol? How much alcohol is usually consumed in a day/week? Has the patient ever had withdrawal symptoms? Has the patient ever been to an alcohol treatment program? What is the patient's current mental status? What is the patient's nutritional status? What is the skin's integrity?

c.   One nursing diagnosis is *Chronic Low Self-Esteem* (©2012 NANDA-I) related to substance abuse. The patient outcome is stable self-esteem. A second nursing diagnosis is *Compromised Family Coping* (©2012 NANDA-I) related to substance abuse. The patient outcome is the family will understand the behaviors needed to support a drug-free family environment and cope with the recovery process. A third nursing diagnosis is *Risk for Violence* (©2012 NANDA-I) related to altered perceptions and poor impulse control. The patient outcome is no violence experienced; altered perceptions are prevented or treated early. A final nursing diagnosis is *Deficient Knowledge* (©2012 NANDA-I) related to lack of understanding of the use and abuse of alcohol. The patient outcome is the patient will express the causes and treatment of addictions and will be able to express the prevention behaviors necessary to be drug free.

Chapter 12

1.   influenza, tuberculosis, cholera, HIV
2.   Strategic National Stockpile (SNS)
3.   Push packages
4.   protective antibodies
5.   atropine
6.   3 to 4

7. a	8. c	9. b	10. b	11. a	12. c
13. b	14. a	15. b	16. d	17. c	18. e
19. e	20. b	21. d	22. c	23. b	24. f
25. e	26. g	27. d	28. h	29. i	30. a
31. c	32. a	33. d	34. b	35. b	36. b
37. c	38. c	39. d	40. a		

41.   a.   Because the patient has not been exposed to anthrax, antibiotic use is not recommended. The antibiotic is expensive, can cause significant side effects, and, most importantly, can promote the development of bacterial strains that are resistant to antibiotics.

b.   Anthrax vaccine is available. It takes 18 months to complete the six injections. At this point, the CDC recommends vaccination only for laboratory personnel who work with anthrax, military personnel in high-risk areas, and those who deal with animal products imported from areas where the disease is endemic.

42.   a.   Assessments include checking for history of eczema, atopic dermatitis, and other exfoliative skin conditions, or patients who have the disease at present; checking for an alteration in immunity (HIV, AIDS, leukemia, lymphoma, immunosuppressive drugs); pregnancy or breast-feeding; age of the patient; and

previous allergic reaction to any component of the vaccine.

b.   Information included in a pamphlet should include:

1.   The vaccine provides high-level protection if given prior to exposure or up to 3 days later.
2.   Protection may last from 3 to 5 years.
3.   The vaccine is contraindicated in people with serious skin conditions, immunocompromised persons, pregnant or lactating women, children under the age of 1 year, and anyone allergic to its components *unless* there is a documented face-to-face contact with an infected person.
4.   This vaccine is known for serious side effects. Of every million people vaccinated, 250 could die from the vaccine.

43.   a.   Potassium iodide prevents damage to the thyroid gland *only* after radiation exposure. It *does not* protect any other body tissues. It will not prevent radiation sickness or other cancers that may develop as a result of the exposure.

b.   Potassium iodide will be absorbed by the thyroid gland and prevent the radioactive iodine from being absorbed by the gland. This lessens the gland's exposure to radiation and prevents the cancer. KI is effective even if taken 3 to 4 hours after exposure.

Chapter 13

1.   central, peripheral
2.   autonomic
3.   fight-or-flight, rest-and-digest
4.   Norepinephrine, acetylcholine
5.   adrenergic, cholinergic
6.   parasympathetic, sympathetic
7.   Adrenergic antagonists
8.   adrenergic (or sympathetic)
9.   Cholinergic

10. e	11. b	12. c	13. d	14. a	15. c
16. b	17. a	18. e	19. d	20. b	21. c
22. a	23. d	24. c	25. d	26. a	27. a
28. d	29. a	30. a	31. c	32. a	33. b
34. b	35. a	36. b	37. a	38. c	39. a
40. c	41. a	42. a	43. d	44. c	

45. $\dfrac{20\ mg}{1} \times \dfrac{5\ cc}{10\ mg} = \dfrac{100}{10} = 10\ cc$

$\dfrac{10\ cc}{dose} \times 4\ doses = 40\ cc/day$

46. $\dfrac{0.3\ mg}{1} \times \dfrac{1\ mL}{0.6\ mg} = \dfrac{0.3}{0.6} = 0.5\ mL$

47.

Drug	Class	Effect or Action	Interactions	
Benadryl	Anticholinergic	Dries secretions causing difficulty for clients with COPD	Increases heart rate and blood pressure	Causes drowsiness Urinary hesitancy and retention
Propranolol	Adrenergic blocker	Decreases bronchodilation causing difficulty for COPD clients	Decreases heart rate and blood pressure Causes orthostatic hypotension	Causes drowsiness and possible depression
Prazosin	Adrenergic blocker	Decreases bronchodilation causing difficulty for COPD clients	Vasodilation to decrease BP, allows increased heart rate	Urinary hesitancy
Proventil	Adrenergic	Bronchodilation	Increases BP and HR	

These actions work against each other in the cardiovascular areas and respiratory areas.

a. Potential nursing diagnoses would include:

1. *Ineffective Airway Clearance* (©2012 NANDA-I) due to drying of secretions caused by Benadryl and interference with bronchodilation when propranolol is given with albuterol

2. Possible *Altered Urinary Elimination: Retention or Hesitancy* (©2012 NANDA-I) related to use of prazosin and Benadryl

3. Possible *Altered Cardiac Output: Decrease* (©2012 NANDA-I) related to use of prazosin, propranolol

b. Nursing interventions that can be done to decrease possible problems or interactions include:

1. Identify interactions and review with the health care provider when appropriate.

2. Increase hydration to 3 L/day to decrease risk of drying of secretions causing altered airway clearance.

3. Monitor for signs of orthostatic hypotension, and possible decreases or increases in blood pressure or pulse.

4. Monitor intake and output to be sure patient maintains urine output and experiences no urinary dysfunction due to adverse medication effects.

48. a. To identify a nursing diagnosis, the nurse would assess the following:

1. Muscle strength
2. Knowledge of the medication regimen
3. Compliance with medication regimen
4. Unusual activities of daily living
5. Unusual medical conditions
6. Previous medications and present medications
7. Administration of medications

b. Nursing diagnoses would include the following:

1. *Risk for Injury* (©2012 NANDA-I)
2. *Impaired Physical Mobility* (©2012 NANDA-I)
3. *Deficient Knowledge* (©2012 NANDA-I)

c. Nursing interventions would include the following:

1. Impaired physical mobility: Assess for muscle strength and neuro status

2. Risk for injury: Assist for need for assistance with mobility; monitor for proper use of mobility equipment: canes, walkers, and transfers; monitor for safety hazards in home; monitor for ability to chew and swallow

3. Deficient Knowledge: Monitor for patient's knowledge before and after teaching about medications, and safety teaching

Chapter 14

1. generalized anxiety disorder (GAD)
2. limbic, reticular activating
3. Anxiolytics, hypnotics
4. GABA receptor–chloride
5. benzodiazepines
6. Barbiturates
7. Respiratory depression
8. IV, III
9. Antidepressants
10. b   11. a   12. c   13. e   14. d   15. d
16. f   17. b   18. a   19. c   20. e   21. b
22. d   23. a   24. d   25. c   26. d   27. c

28. a   29. d   30. b   31. b   32. b   33. c
34. b   35. b   36. b   37. d   38. d   39. a

40. $\dfrac{1.5 \text{ mg}}{\text{dose}} \times \dfrac{1 \text{ g}}{1,000 \text{ mg}} \times \dfrac{1 \text{ mL}}{0.001 \text{ g}} = \dfrac{1.5}{1} = \dfrac{1.5 \text{ mL}}{\text{dose}}$

41. $\dfrac{1 \text{ mg}}{\text{dose}} \times \dfrac{1 \text{ mL}}{5 \text{ mg}} = \dfrac{1}{5} = \dfrac{0.2 \text{ mL}}{\text{dose}}$

42. a. Nursing assessments prior to giving Versed include:
    1. Allergies to benzodiazepines or chemically similar drugs
    2. Liver and renal function
    3. History of any chronic respiratory conditions
    4. History of depression, alcohol or drug abuse
    5. Medications taken routinely and when taken last, including herbals

    b. Nursing interventions would include:
    1. Resuscitation equipment, and airway
    2. Romazicon as benzodiazepine blocker
    3. Ventilator
    4. Someone to take patient home after the procedure
    5. Monitor vital signs every 5–15 min, especially respiratory rate and depth
    6. Monitor patient's level of consciousness and responsiveness

    c. To evaluate the effectiveness of intervention, the nurse would use the following:
    1. The patient has no injury related to the administration of Versed.
    2. The patient has normal vital signs during the administration of Versed.

43. a. *Sleep Pattern Disturbance* (©2012 NANDA-I) related to anxiety response

    b. Interventions include:
    1. Explore potential contributing factors
    2. Maintain bedtime routine as per patient preference
    3. Provide comfort measures to induce sleep:
       a. Nonpharmacologic techniques
       b. Back rub
       c. Light bedtime snack
       d. Establish a regular time to sleep
       e. Avoid napping during the day
       f. Decrease caffeine, chocolate, nicotine, and other stimulants in the second half of the day
       g. Limit alcohol consumption
       h. Exercise at least 2–3 hours before bedtime
       i. Hot bath 1 hour before sleep
       j. Comfortable sleeping environment
       k. Use stress reduction and relaxation just prior to sleep
       l. Relief of pain or discomfort prior to sleep

    c. Pharmacologic techniques will provide information to patient regarding pharmacotherapeutics. Benzodiazepines would be the drug of first choice for sleep. However, all of these drugs will cause interruption of REM sleep and, therefore, should not be continued for more than 1 week. Certain over-the-counter drugs are normally anticholinergics and also interrupt REM sleep, can cause a hangover, and should not be used for more than 1 week.

Chapter 15

1. seizure
2. infections, trauma, metabolic disorders, vascular diseases, pediatric disorders, neoplastic disease
3. contraceptive measures
4. folate
5. sleep, strobe, flickering
6. Febrile, 3, 5, fever (or temperature)
7. carbamazepine (Tegretol)
8. Partial, complete
9. ethosuximide (Zarontin)
10. diazepam (Valium), phenytoin (Dilantin)
11. Status epilepticus, respirations (or breathing)
12. airway
13. abnormal, suppress
14. 3, months

15. f	16. e	17. b	18. a	19. c	20. g
21. d	22. d	23. a	24. b	25. a	26. b
27. c	28. d	29. c	30. b	31. b	32. a
33. d	34. a	35. d	36. d	37. c	38. b
39. a	40. b	41. d	42. c	43. c	44. a
45. a					

46. $\dfrac{60 \text{ mg}}{\text{dose}} \times \dfrac{5 \text{ mL}}{20 \text{ mg}} = \dfrac{300}{20} = \dfrac{15 \text{ mL}}{\text{dose}}$

47. $\dfrac{1,200 \text{ mg}}{4 \text{ doses}} = 300 \text{ mg/dose}$

48. a. Possible risk of injury related to medication administration: Inappropriate administration of Dilantin IV can lead to emboli, hypoventilation, hypotension, venous irritation, seizures, or decreased level of consciousness.

    b. Nursing interventions for administration of Dilantin IV:
    1. Use saline only to mix Dilantin.
    2. Infuse no faster than 50 mg/min.
    3. Use IV line with filter.
    4. Check for infiltration often, as it is a soft tissue irritant.

5. Use large vein or central venous catheter only.

6. Never use Dilantin IM.

7. Avoid hand veins to prevent local vasoconstriction.

8. Prime IV line with saline if hanging piggyback.

9. Monitor for LOC changes after seizure.

10. Keep side rails up and padded.

11. Have emergency equipment available.

12. Monitor for hypotension or depressed respirations during administration.

49. a. Top priority diagnosis: *Deficient Knowledge* (©2012 NANDA-I) related to new medical condition and new medication for management of seizures as evidenced by patient asking questions

   b. Interventions:

   1. Assess what the patient knows about epilepsy, seizures, and management.

   2. Assess for any misunderstandings about medication and treatment regimen.

   3. Provide information to patient regarding the following:

      a. Medications will be dosed at the lowest dosage to prevent seizures, which will decrease the amount of side effects expected.

      b. The medication dosages will be increased as needed if seizures continue.

      c. Other medications might be added or drugs might be changed as needed to control seizures.

   4. Seizures will be controlled best if patients are compliant with the medication schedule. Patients will need to return for lab appointments and follow-up health care provider visit to evaluate therapeutic effect.

   5. Side effects that might be expected initially include dizziness, ataxia, diplopia, and a change of urine color to pink, red, or brown. The dizziness and drowsiness will decrease as the medication is continued.

   6. More serious side effects should be reported to the health care provider.

   7. Drugs to avoid: Many medications interact with phenytoin. The patient must inform the health care provider that he is on phenytoin before any medications are added. The pharmacist might also be consulted before over-the-counter medications and herbals or supplements are added.

   8. No foods need to be avoided, but supplements of folic acid, calcium, and vitamin D will impair the Dilantin. The nurse should give the patient a list of foods that contain folic acid, calcium, and vitamin D. These foods should not be taken in large quantities, although they do not need to be avoided.

Chapter 16

1. seasonal affective disorder

2. major depressive disorder, bipolar disorder

3. tricyclic antidepressants (TCAs), selective serotonin reuptake inhibitors (SSRIs), monoamine oxidase inhibitors (MAOIs)

4. SSRIs

5. TCAs

6. lithium

7. attention deficit/hyperactivity disorder (ADHD)

8. CNS stimulants

9. mood stabilizers, mania, depression

10. f	11. e	12. d	13. b	14. c	15. a
16. a	17. c	18. b	19. e	20. d	21. d
22. c	23. e	24. b	25. a	26. d	27. b
28. d	29. d	30. a	31. d	32. d	33. c
34. c	35. b	36. d	37. b	38. a	39. c
40. b	41. d	42. c	43. a	44. b	45. a
46. d					

47. $\dfrac{1.2\ g}{day}\times\dfrac{1{,}000\ mg}{1\ g}\times\dfrac{1\ capsule}{300\ mg}=\dfrac{1{,}200}{300}=4\ capsules$

$\dfrac{4\ capsules}{4\ doses}=\dfrac{1\ capsule}{dose}$

48. $\dfrac{45\ mg}{day}\times\dfrac{5\ mL}{20\ mg}=\dfrac{225}{20}=\dfrac{11.25\ mL}{day}$

49. a. *Risk for Injury* (©2012 NANDA-I) related to adverse effects of lithium

   b. The nurse should assess for the following:

   1. Knowledge of side effects: Dizziness, drowsiness, nausea, metallic taste, tremors, vomiting, and diarrhea

   2. Lab studies: Renal and kidney function, blood levels of lithium

   3. Interactions: Diuretics and low-sodium diet possibly leading to lithium toxicity

   4. History: Allergies or previous renal or cardiac conditions

   5. Mental and emotional status: Previous suicide attempts or present intent

   6. Knowledge of whom to notify in case of adverse or toxic effects of lithium

   7. Knowledge of adverse and toxic effects of lithium

   c. The goal is to demonstrate the following:

   1. Understanding of drug effects and precautions

   2. Improvement in mood stability

   3. Ability to notify or seek help when questions or problems arise

   4. No injury related to adverse effects of lithium

50.

Goals for the Patient	Evaluation
Patient will show (or report):	
Improved affect or mood	No longer has suicidal ideation
	Engages in normal daily activities
Improved sleep patterns	Can sleep through the night, stays asleep, and falls asleep easily
Decreasing episodes of side effects	Decreased headaches, of side effects nausea, drowsiness since beginning medications
Continuation of medication regimen	Continues to take medications as ordered

Chapter 17

1. schizophrenia
2. hours to days, months to years
3. positive, negative
4. genetic component, imbalances in neurotransmitters
5. hallucinations, delusions, disorganized thoughts, disorganized speech patterns
6. interest, motivation, responsiveness, pleasure
7. antipsychotic
8. dopamine (D_2)
9. schizophrenia, extrapyramidal
10. b 11. a 12. a 13. a 14. c 15. a
16. c 17. d 18. b 19. c 20. f 21. b
22. d 23. g 24. a 25. e 26. c 27. h
28. i 29. b 30. c 31. d 32. b 33. d
34. b 35. b 36. c 37. b 38. a 39. c
40. a 41. c 42. d 43. d

44. $\dfrac{15 \text{ mg}}{\text{dose}} \times \dfrac{1 \text{ mL}}{25 \text{ mg}} = \dfrac{15}{25} = \dfrac{0.6 \text{ mL}}{\text{dose}}$

45. $\dfrac{200 \text{ mg}}{\text{day}} \times \dfrac{1 \text{ tablet}}{50 \text{ mg}} = \dfrac{200}{50} = \dfrac{4 \text{ tablets}}{\text{day}}$

$\dfrac{4 \text{ tablets}}{2 \text{ doses}} = \dfrac{2 \text{ tablets}}{\text{dose}}$

46. a. Interventions used for the diagnosis of *Deficient Knowledge* (©2012 NANDA-I):
   1. Assess patient's readiness to learn based on his or her emotional response.
   2. Provide health teaching related to Clozaril:
      a. Can cause drowsiness, dry mouth, and hypotension.
      b. Does not cause as many problems with EPS as Thorazine does.
      c. Get up slowly to prevent dizziness and falls due to orthostatic hypotension.
      d. Avoid activities requiring mental alertness until effects of medication are known.
      e. Avoid alcohol and other CNS depressants.
      f. Weekly labs are required to monitor for agranulocytosis.
      g. Report any evidence of infection: sore throat and mild fever.
   3. Instruct patient on best time to take the medication and what to do for missed doses.
   b. Evaluation will include the following:
      1. The patient will report to lab and health care provider for appointments as requested for lab work.
      2. The patient will not experience injury (falls) related to dizziness, sedation, or ataxia.
      3. The patient remains compliant with therapeutic regimen prescribed.
      4. The patient verbalizes understanding of medical regimen, adverse effects of medication, and the need to be compliant.

47. Assessments include the following:
   1. Assess vital signs: temp, pulse, blood pressure, and body weight.
   2. Assess behavior and appearances: dietary intake, activities of daily living, and socialization with others.
   3. Assess the symptoms of the condition: hallucinations, delusions, enjoyment of life, personal hygiene, speech patterns, and motor movement.
   4. Monitor for side effects and adverse effects of medications such as akathisia, abnormal movements, dizziness, drowsiness, constipation, photosensitivity, or orthostatic hypotension.
   5. Let patient know that side effects will decrease with time on the medication.
   6. Assess any past history of seizures; medication can influence the seizure threshold.
   7. Assess plans for pregnancy or if any contraceptives are being used.
   8. Monitor for fluid volume deficit by monitoring intake and output, and weight, daily. Teach patient to increase oral intake to maintain hydration.
   9. Monitor for improvement in symptoms of condition. Worsening of the condition should be reported immediately.
   10. Monitor compliance with medication regimen.
   11. Assess present medications or herbs that may interact with the new medication.

Chapter 18

1. opioid (narcotic), nonopioid (nonnarcotic)
2. anti-inflammatory, antipyretic
3. tension

4. aura

5. nociceptor (peripheral tissue)

6. anxiety, depression, fatigue

7. characteristic, nature

8. stop, prevent

9. triptans, ergot alkaloids, serotonin

10. intracranial vessels, orally, parenterally, nasally

11. d	12. c	13. a	14. b	15. e	16. d
17. a	18. e	19. c	20. a	21. e	22. e
23. f	24. d	25. a	26. c	27. b	28. e
29. a	30. c	31. c	32. d	33. b	34. a
35. c	36. d	37. a	38. d	39. a	40. b
41. c	42. c	43. b	44. d	45. b	46. c
47. a	48. c				

49. $\dfrac{400 \text{ mg}}{\text{dose}} \times \dfrac{5 \text{ mL}}{100 \text{ mg}} = \dfrac{2000}{100} = \dfrac{20 \text{ mL}}{\text{dose}}$

50. $\dfrac{0.4 \text{ mg}}{\text{dose}} \times \dfrac{1 \text{ mL}}{0.02 \text{ mg}} = \dfrac{0.4}{0.02} = \dfrac{20 \text{ mL}}{\text{dose}}$

51. a. Interventions include:

1. Assess the psychosocial situation of the patient because anxiety, fatigue, and pain will increase the sensation of pain.

2. Analyze the cultural aspects of the patient's pain.

3. Assess the knowledge of the patient about addiction and use of narcotic analgesics.

4. Teach the patient nonpharmacologic aspects of pain control: relaxation, massage, thermal packs, or biofeedback.

5. Discuss the source of pain and the therapeutic management for the patient's pain, including using narcotic pain reliever only after less potent medications are attempted first.

6. Teach the patient to assess levels of pain with objective methods to quantify pain in order to better evaluate management of pain.

7. Teach the patient to journal to identify triggers for the pain.

b. The outcome is that the patient will report less pain after interventions and more relief from both pharmacologic and nonpharmacologic pain management techniques.

52. a. Interventions include:

1. Assess the patient's medication regimen.

2. Educate the patient on possible nonpharmacologic approaches: relaxation, biofeedback, massage, or thermal therapy.

3. Educate the patient on triggers that can cause migraines. Help the patient identify triggers that might apply.

4. Teach the patient appropriate administration techniques of the medications:

   a. Take Percodan as aura begins and do not wait until headache is severe.

b. Teach the patient to evaluate the level of pain and evaluate the improvement using pain scale of choice.

5. Encourage the patient to revisit the health care provider if no improvement has been made with present medications. Encourage the patient to request or ask if additional medications might be helpful.

b. Goals include the following:

1. Patient will identify triggers to migraines and eliminate the triggers.

2. Patient will gain comfort by using nonpharmacologic approaches to migraine discomfort.

3. Patient will identify a decrease in discomfort after medication is taken.

4. Empower the patient to seek medication or measures in addition to those previously named.

Chapter 19

1. surface (or regional)

2. infiltration (or field block)

3. consciousness

4. IV, inhaled

5. pain following surgery

6. sensations, consciousness

7. location, extent of desired anesthesias

8. sensation, muscle activity

9. anticholinergic, benzodiazepine, cholinergic, dopamine blocker, neuromuscular blockers, opioids, phenothiazine

10. balanced, lowered

11. e	12. a	13. b	14. c	15. d	16. b
17. b	18. d, e	19. e	20. d	21. c	22. d, e
23. d	24. a	25. d	26. e	27. b	28. e
29. c	30. h	31. g	32. f	33. d	34. d
35. a	36. b	37. c	38. d	39. c	40. b
41. c	42. a	43. a	44. d	45. b	46. b
47. d	48. a	49. b	50. b		

51. $\dfrac{\frac{1}{6}\text{gr}}{\text{dose}} \times \dfrac{1}{1 \text{ gr}} \times \dfrac{1 \text{ mL}}{15 \text{ mg}} = \dfrac{\frac{60}{6}}{15} = \dfrac{10}{15} = \dfrac{0.67 \text{ mL}}{\text{dose}}$

52. $\dfrac{100 \text{ mg}}{\text{dose}} \times \dfrac{2 \text{ cc}}{200 \text{ mg}} = \dfrac{200}{200} = \dfrac{1 \text{ mL}}{\text{dose}}$

53. a. *Deficient Knowledge* (©2012 NANDA-I) related to upcoming surgery and unknown medication regimen

b. Interventions include preoperative surgical preparation and teaching:

1. Preoperative medications are given to relieve anxiety and provide sedation.

2. Anticholinergics are given to dry secretions to prevent pneumonia and aspiration.

3. Pain medications are given to aid in pain control.

4. An IV medication is given to cause rapid unconsciousness.

5. After IV medications take effect, the patient is given an inhaled anesthesia.

6. Muscle relaxants are given to provide relaxation, during which time the patient will breathe with use of a ventilator.

7. Postoperative medications will include analgesics for the patient, and antiemetics if needed to prevent vomiting.

8. Assess the patient's understanding of the information given.

9. Ask if the patient has any questions.

54. a. The nursing diagnosis is *Anxiety* (©2012 NANDA-I) related to anticipated pain of invasive procedure as evidenced by inability to concentrate; appearance of nervousness, apprehension, and tension; restlessness; and hyperattentiveness.

b. Assessment data include rapid pressured speech, tremulousness, restlessness, scanning of room, and asking questions.

c. Interventions are as follows:

1. Assist patient to reduce level of anxiety by reassurance and staying with the patient.

2. Speak slowly and calmly when giving information.

3. Ask about any physical problems and past history as well as present medications.

4. Give clear, concise information when teaching about the medications to be used.

5. Discuss alternate methods of relaxation.

6. Help establish short-term goals and reinforce positive responses to questions and actions.

7. Initiate health teaching in short, concise statements and move at the patient's own rate.

8. Monitor vital signs and any evidence of shortness of breath or chest pain.

d. Goals for the patient may include the following:

1. The patient will demonstrate a decrease in anxiety as shown by slower speech patterns, decreased vital signs, and the ability to repeat instruction-and-answer questions in a focused method.

2. The patient will relate information offered during the teaching session relating to the upcoming procedure.

3. The patient will relate information that has been taught throughout the teaching session.

e. Vital signs are normal. The patient repeats instructions and answers questions appropriately.

Chapter 20

1. dopamine, acetylcholine
2. Alzheimer's disease
3. unknown
4. acetylcholine
5. genetic
6. antipsychotic, extrapyramidal
7. hypotension, tachycardia; muscle twitching, mood changes
8. cognitive, behavioral, activities of daily living (ADLs)
9. acetylcholinesterase inhibitors, functioning
10. b 11. a 12. c 13. a 14. b 15. c
16. a 17. a 18. b 19. c 20. i 21. h
22. g 23. e 24. f 25. a 26. c 27. d
28. b 29. a 30. d 31. d 32. a 33. a
34. c 35. a 36. b 37. a 38. d 39. c
40. c 41. a 42. c 43. b 44. d 45. b
46. a

47.
$$\frac{100 \text{ mg}}{\text{dose}} \times \frac{1 \text{ tablet}}{25 \text{ mg}} = \frac{100}{25} = \frac{4 \text{ tablets}}{\text{dose}}$$

$$\frac{4 \text{ tablets}}{\text{dose}} \times \frac{3 \text{ doses}}{1} = \frac{12 \text{ tablets}}{\text{day}}$$

48.
$$\frac{7.5 \text{ mg}}{3 \text{ doses}} = \frac{2.5 \text{ mg}}{\text{dose}}$$

49. a. The nursing diagnosis is *Risk for Injury* (©2012 NANDA-I) related to drug effects and unresolved symptoms of parkinsonism. This diagnosis relates to sedation as a side effect of anticholinergics and of interactions with other possible CNS depressants such as Zoloft. The tremors and involuntary movements also cause possible balance problems. Orthostatic hypotension is also a side effect that causes balance instability.

b. The patient will have no injury related to the side effects of medications or the condition (Parkinson's disease).

50. a. The priority diagnosis at this point would be *Risk of Injury* (©2012 NANDA-I) related to possible adverse effects of drugs and interactions.

b. Interventions would include:

1. Assess for interactions between medications in the regimen.

2. Tricyclics and benzodiazepines can potentiate their CNS depression, causing sedation and sleep deprivation.

3. Assess for side effects of the medications:

a. Sedation, vomiting, diarrhea, obstructed urine flow, insomnia, abnormal dreaming, aggression, syncope, depression, headache, irritability, fatigue, urinary incontinence, and restlessness

4. Provide instructions for proper administration:

a. Give at bedtime and once daily.

b. Maintain a regular medication schedule.

c. Provide assistance to the patient when memory is impaired.

5. Assess for contraindicated conditions or medications:

a. Hypotension, bradycardia, hyperthyroid, peptic ulcer disease

6. Teach safety precautions for side effects of medications: no hot showers, arise slowly, have something to hold on to during ambulation when needed.

7. Include family and patient in management of the patient's condition.

8. Collaborate with other departments as needed: PT, OT, home health care.

9. Assess for caregiver strain.

10. Monitor for improvement with the patient's short-term memory or behaviors while on medications.

Chapter 21

1. movement
2. nervous, muscular, endocrine, skeletal
3. muscle spasms
4. analgesics, anti-inflammatory agents, antispasmodic
5. spasticity
6. dystonia
7. tonic spasms

8. a   9. b   10. b   11. a   12. a   13. b
14. a   15. a   16. b   17. a   18. b   19. d
20. b   21. c   22. a   23. d   24. b   25. a
26. c   27. b   28. a   29. d   30. b   31. b
32. b

33. $\dfrac{75 \text{ mg}}{\text{dose}} \times \dfrac{1 \text{ tablet}}{25 \text{ mg}} = \dfrac{75}{25} = \dfrac{3 \text{ tablets}}{\text{dose}}$

$\dfrac{75 \text{ mg}}{\text{dose}} \times \dfrac{2 \text{ doses}}{\text{day}} = \dfrac{150 \text{ mg}}{\text{day}}$

34. $\dfrac{20 \text{ mg}}{\text{dose}} \times \dfrac{1 \text{ tablet}}{10 \text{ mg}} = \dfrac{20}{10} = \dfrac{2 \text{ tablets}}{\text{dose}}$

Yes—safe dose.

35. a. Limiting use of the affected muscle, heat or cold packs, hydrotherapy, ultrasound, exercises, massage, and manipulation may help to decrease the patient's low back pain.

b. The patient needs to know that dizziness, dry mouth, rash, and a fast pulse rate with palpitations may be noted while using this drug. Another possible but rare reaction is swelling of the tongue. She should not take this drug with alcohol, phenothiazines, or MAO inhibitors because of unfavorable reactions.

c. Ask the patient to rate her pain on a scale of 1 to 10 and see whether improvement is noted after using the drug. Monitor muscle tone, ROM, and improved ability to do ADLs. These should increase if the drug is effective.

d. The patient should be instructed in proper body mechanics while lifting, sitting, or engaged in other musculoskeletal movement activities.

36. a. The patient needs to know that Botox injections are indicated for moderate to severe frown lines.

They are not for crow's feet. She also needs to know that they will, however, smooth the lines between the brows temporarily, and must be repeated every 3 to 4 months. Although botulinum toxin is a poison in higher quantities, it is safe for use in tiny injections.

b. Side effects of Botox include headache, nausea, flulike symptoms, temporary blepharoptosis, mild pain, erythema at the site of injection, and muscle weakness.

37. a. The patient should have a thorough assessment of his physical condition, especially vital signs, skin condition, mobility or lack of mobility, neurologic function, self-care ability, and nutritional status. The nurse should also determine the adherence to his medication regimen, side effects, and what outcome the family expects.

b. Physical therapy exercises might decrease the severity of his symptoms. These include stretching to help prevent contractures, muscle-group strengthening exercises, and repetitive motion exercises. Surgery for tendon release or to sever the nerve–muscle pathway might be used in an extreme situation.

c. The patient and his family should be instructed to report any significant changes in his level of consciousness such as confusion, hallucinations, lethargy, and decreased speech ability. Also, palpitations, chest pain, dyspnea, visual disturbances, and unusual fatigue should be reported to the health care provider. Treatment should not be discontinued abruptly. Taking the medications with food should decrease GI upset. Decreased urinary output, distended abdomen, and discomfort should be reported. Dry mouth may be treated with sips of water, sugarless candy, or gum if patient is able to use this.

d. The family/patient need to be instructed on gentle ROM and other physical therapy as indicated by the health care provider. Safety measures include rearranging the home to decrease the risk of falls or accidents, and placing needed objects within the patient's reach.

Chapter 22

1. hyperlipidemia
2. plaque
3. triglycerides, phospholipids, steroids
4. cholesterol, triglycerides, phospholipids
5. statin

6. b   7. d   8. c   9. a   10. c   11. b
12. b   13. d   14. d   15. d   16. b   17. b
18. a   19. d   20. c   21. b   22. c   23. a
24. c   25. c

26. $\dfrac{40 \text{ mg}}{1} \times \dfrac{1 \text{ tablet}}{20 \text{ mg}} = \dfrac{40}{20} = 2 \text{ tablets}$

27. 2 tablets, divide the dose, give one in the morning 30 minutes before breakfast, and 1 tablet 30 minutes before the evening meal

$$\frac{1.2\ g}{1} \times \frac{1{,}000\ mg}{1\ g} \times \frac{1\ tablet}{600\ mg} = \frac{1{,}200}{600} = 2\ tablets$$

28. a. Data assessment includes obesity; history of two heart attacks; history of hypertension, elevated LDL, and elevated triglycerides.

   b. Therapy with a statin drug is highly indicated because the patient has a history of heart disease and hypertension with elevated lipid levels.

   c. Reduce dietary intake of lipids and explain exercise program.

29. a. Ascertain if the patient is taking the drugs as prescribed. If she is taking the drugs, then dietary habit changes are important to discuss, especially lipid-rich foods. Many patients believe that if they are taking lipid-lowering agents, they do not have to watch their dietary fat intake.

   b. Teach risk factor modification, which includes diet restrictions related to fats, calorie assessment, exercise assessment, stress assessment, knowledge, and understanding of when to take statin drugs. Remember that it is best to take some of the statin drugs in the evening, because the body produces the most cholesterol during the night.

Chapter 23

1. distal
2. distal, reabsorbed, secreted
3. A. efferent arteriole
   B. peritubular capillaries
   C. proximal tubule
   D. distal tubule
   E. collecting duct
   F. loop of Henle
   G. Bowman's capsule
   H. glomerulus
   I. afferent arteriole
4. a   5. b   6. c   7. b   8. e   9. c
10. d   11. a   12. c   13. b   14. b   15. a
16. d   17. c   18. d   19. a   20. b   21. c
22. b   23. d   24. a   25. c   26. a   27. d
28. a   29. d   30. d   31. b   32. d

33. $$\frac{1\ mg}{dose} \times \frac{1\ tablet}{0.5\ mg} = \frac{1.0}{0.5} = \frac{2\ tablets}{dose}$$

34. $$\frac{100\ mL}{2\ h} \times \frac{10\ gtt}{1\ mL} \times \frac{1\ h}{60\ min} = \frac{1{,}000}{120}$$
$$= \frac{8.33\ gtt}{min} = \frac{8\ gtt}{min}$$

35. a. Nursing diagnoses may include *Risk for Injury*, *Fatigue*, and *Deficient Knowledge* (©2012 NANDA-I).

   b. The nurse needs to monitor blood pressure and ask the patient for recent blood pressure values. Inquire about the patient's medication regimen. Review serum potassium levels. Obtain more information about presenting symptoms such as onset, alleviating and aggravating factors, and intensity. Inquire about other symptoms of hyperkalemia including irritability, anxiety, and abdominal cramping. Obtain a 24-hour nutrition history including beverages.

36. a. It is important for the nurse to communicate to the patient the health complications related to untreated hypertension. Assessment of the patient's lifestyle and stressors is also vital information needed to create an adequate plan of care.

   b. Lifestyle activities to reduce blood pressure should be communicated to the patient. Many factors may contribute to high blood pressure. These factors are often difficult to manage and most patients require assistance to make the changes necessary to improve their health. The patient should be advised of the health hazards related to smoking, lack of exercise, obesity, stress, and alcohol consumption. The nurse should choose teaching methods appropriate for the patient's busy lifestyle. Handouts and written material will reinforce teaching and allow the patient to refer to the information at a later date. Follow-up appointments can be used to document progress in making lifestyle changes. Support groups may provide the patient with encouragement and accountability.

Chapter 24

1. Crystalloids
2. 7.35
3. 7.35 to 7.45
4. decrease
5. Hypertonic
6. Hypotonic
7. Isotonic
8. a   9. b   10. b   11. a   12. b   13. d
14. b   15. b   16. a   17. d   18. b   19. a
20. d   21. c   22. a   23. c   24. a   25. c
26. a   27. c   28. d   29. a   30. b

31. $$\frac{1{,}000\ mL}{8\ h} = \frac{125\ mL}{h}$$

32. $$\frac{8\ g}{day} \times \frac{1{,}000\ mg}{1\ g} \times \frac{1\ tablet}{500\ mg} = \frac{8{,}000}{500} = \frac{16\ tablets}{day}$$
$$\frac{16\ tablets}{4\ doses} = \frac{4\ tablets}{dose}$$

33. a. Aspirin and potassium may irritate the stomach mucosa. Also, an extremely low carbohydrate diet

causes the body to burn fats for energy, creating ketoacids. CNS depression may be caused by an impending acidosis. The patient has a knowledge deficit of her drug regimen requiring nursing intervention.

b. The patient could benefit from a thorough nutritional assessment and resulting weight loss plan taking her drug regimen into consideration. Referral to a nutritionist may be necessary. The nurse should also ensure that the patient understands proper administration of her drug regimen.

34. a. Symptoms of hyponatremia include nausea, vomiting, muscle cramps, tachycardia, dry mucous membranes, and headache. The nurse should obtain a baseline set of vital signs and monitor values closely. The patient should be asked about the onset and progression of symptoms. A diet history including beverages should be obtained.

b. A hazard of working outdoors is sodium loss through profuse sweating. Fluid replacement is critical to avoid hyponatremia. The nurse should encourage the patient to consume adequate amounts of water or electrolyte solutions such as sports drinks. The early symptoms of hyponatremia should serve as a signal to take refuge from the heat and concentrate on fluid replacement.

Chapter 25

1. primary (or idiopathic or essential) hypertension
2. increasing peripheral resistance
3. relax (dilate), decreasing
4. angiotensin II, aldosterone
5. Reflex tachycardia
6. fight-or-flight
7. Diuretics
8. f   9. c   10. a   11. c   12. b   13. c
14. g   15. d   16. a   17. b   18. d   19. c
20. a   21. c   22. d   23. a   24. a   25. b
26. c   27. c   28. a   29. b   30. a   31. d
32. a   33. c   34. c   35. d   36. a

37. $\dfrac{15 \text{ mg}}{1} \times \dfrac{2 \text{ mL}}{20 \text{ mg}} = 1.5 \text{ mL}$

38. $\dfrac{60 \text{ mg}}{1} \times \dfrac{1 \text{ tablet}}{120 \text{ mg}} = \frac{1}{2} \text{ tablet}$

39. a. Assessment data include smoking, overweight, elevated lipids, and anxiety.

b. Nursing diagnoses are as follows:

1. *Imbalanced Nutrition: More than Body Requirements* (©2012 NANDA-I) (Outcome: Patient demonstrates accurate knowledge of dietary regimen to lower dietary fats.)

2. *Deficient Knowledge*: (©2012 NANDA-I) Purpose, precautions, and side effects of antihypertensive drugs (Outcome: Patient will verbalize accurate understanding of the purpose, precautions, and side effects of drugs used to treat hypertension.)

3. *Health-Seeking Behaviors*: (©2012 NANDA-I) Relaxation techniques to effectively reduce stress (Outcome: Patient reports subjective relief of stress after using relaxation techniques.)

c. The health care provider will consider adding a second antihypertensive drug class if the first drug has proven to be inadequate in treatment of HTN. It is common to prescribe drugs from two antihypertensives classes concurrently to manage resistant HTN.

40. a. Orthostatic hypotension may be causing the dizziness. Explaining to the patient that she should sit on the side of the bed a few minutes before standing might solve this problem.

b. Cardiac rhythm abnormalities are one sign of possible hyperkalemia. When switched to a potassium-sparing diuretic such as spironolactone, the patient should not supplement her diet with excess potassium.

c. It may not be necessary to change this patient's medications, because they seem to be keeping blood pressure within normal limits. Patient teaching may be all that is necessary to resolve the patient's complaints.

Chapter 26

1. Frank-Starling
2. 60
3. preload, afterload
4. increase, strength
5. forcefully, slowly
6. digoxin immune Fab (Digibind)
7. calcium
8. c   9. e   10. d   11. a   12. f   13. c
14. b   15. c   16. e   17. d   18. a   19. c
20. d   21. b   22. b   23. c   24. a   25. b
26. a   27. c   28. b   29. c   30. c   31. a
32. d   33. d   34. a   35. c   36. b   37. d
38. a

39. $\dfrac{5 \text{ mcg}}{1 \text{ kg}} \times \dfrac{1}{1 \text{ min}} \times \dfrac{75 \text{ kg}}{1} \times \dfrac{1 \text{ mg}}{1,000 \text{ mcg}} \times \dfrac{40 \text{ mL}}{100 \text{ mg}} \times$

$\dfrac{60 \text{ min}}{1 \text{ hr}} = \dfrac{900,000}{100,000} = \dfrac{9 \text{ mL}}{\text{h}}$

40. $\dfrac{40 \text{ mg}}{1} \times \dfrac{2 \text{ mL}}{20 \text{ mg}} = \dfrac{80}{20} = 4 \text{ mL}$

41. a. Inotropic drugs affect the strength of myocardial contraction; chronotropic drugs affect the heart rate.

b. Cardiac glycosides and the phosphodiesterase inhibitors are examples of drug classes that produce positive inotropic effects. Drugs that stimulate beta$_1$-adrenergic receptors and anticholinergics cause a positive chronotropic response.

c. In heart failure, the nurse wants the heart to eject more blood per contraction; therefore, positive inotropic drugs are needed. Positive chronotropic drugs are useful in treating cardiac failure and cardiogenic shock.

42. a. Hydrochlorothiazide and lisinopril will lower blood pressure, thus reducing the workload on the heart. Atorvastatin will help reduce blood cholesterol levels, which are associated with hypertension and heart disease.

b. The patient is showing a need to control his life and manage his disease. He is 60 years old and he is determined to manage his disease without prescriptions. However, the patient should be encouraged to take the drugs as prescribed. He needs to understand that heart failure is a progressive disorder and that he is in the early stages. He can limit the progression with knowledge and attention to symptoms. He should be advised to try alternative therapies in addition to his medications, not in place of them.

c. The patient should be advised to continue his walks and develop a complete exercise and dietary program, under the direction of his nurse.

43. a. Labored and rapid respirations, coarse breath sounds with wheezing, rapid weight gain, and rapid heart rate support a diagnosis of heart failure.

b. The digoxin is given IV for a fast uptake and action. The 0.5-mg dose with a repeat in 4 hours is considered a loading dose. It is common to give an adult 0.25 mg/day by mouth of digoxin to treat heart failure.

c. This patient needs the renal system evaluated frequently. The output is of extreme importance, as retention of fluid will increase the heart failure. This patient had a 10-lb weight gain in 3 days. The nurse should ask about the hourly urinary output.

Chapter 27

1. angina pectoris
2. plaque
3. stable
4. organic nitrates
5. transdermal patch
6. anticoagulants/antiplatelets

7. c	8. a	9. b	10. b	11. c	12. a
13. c	14. a	15. a	16. c	17. b	18. a
19. d	20. b	21. c	22. c	23. a	24. d
25. a	26. d	27. d	28. b	29. b	30. a
31. c	32. c	33. c	34. c	35. c	36. d
37. d	38. b	39. b	40. a	41. c	

42. $$\frac{50 \text{ mg}}{250 \text{ mL}} \times \frac{1{,}000 \text{ mcg}}{1 \text{ mg}} \times \frac{1 \text{ mL}}{60 \text{ gtt}} \times \frac{15 \text{ gtt}}{1 \text{ min}} =$$

$$\frac{750{,}000}{15{,}000} = \frac{50 \text{ mcg}}{\text{min}}$$

43. $$\frac{100 \text{ mL}}{125 \text{ mg}} \times \frac{60 \text{ gtt}}{1 \text{ mL}} \times \frac{10 \text{ mg}}{1 \text{ h}} \times \frac{1 \text{ h}}{60 \text{ min}} =$$

$$\frac{60{,}000}{7{,}500} = \frac{8 \text{ gtt}}{\text{min}}$$

44. a. The patient's age has put him at risk for atherosclerosis. His heavy tobacco use has predisposed him to vascular disease. His weight has increased the stress on the cardiovascular system. His life may be considered stressful based on the size of his family. He may have led a sedentary life because of his career path as an accountant.

b. Retavase will dissolve the cerebral thrombosis. Lasix will control blood pressure. Heparin prevents further thrombus development.

c. Hydrochlorothiazide is a diuretic that will treat the patient's hypertension. It is a safer drug for home use as it does not lower serum potassium like furosemide (Lasix). Warfarin is taken orally and will be used to provide anticoagulation. This drug is used to prevent further thrombus development and therefore prevent an embolus event. Warfarin is a good discharge anticoagulant because it can be given by mouth. Diltiazem is a calcium channel blocker that is an effective drug to be used at home to stabilize hypertension.

45. a. Nursing diagnoses are as follows:

1. *Altered Tissue Perfusion* (©2012 NANDA-I) related to vascular disease (Outcome: Patient will experience relief of chest pain.)

2. *Pain* (headache) related to adverse effects of medication (Outcome: Patient will experience relief of headaches.)

3. *Decreased Cardiac Output* (©2012 NANDA-I) related to loss of myocardial muscle function (Outcome: Patient has adequate cardiac output within 24 hours of treatment as evidenced by BP $<$160/90 mmHg, respiration $<$ 20/min.)

b. Patient presents with some worsening signs of heart failure. Respiration is elevated to 28/min. Lower extremities are edematous, chest pain is not relieved, and patient is gaining weight.

c. The following reasons may be suspected:

1. Possibly, the patient is not taking the medications correctly. Review the medication delivery systems used to treat her chest pain and determine if she is using the medications correctly.

2. The patient's medical situation may be worsening. Her coronary arteries may be obstructed and cardiac failure is occurring based on coronary occlusion.

3. The patient may be exhibiting tolerance to the nitrates; therefore, new drugs may be necessary to treat her chest pain or current medications may need to be increased in dosage.

4. The combination treatment (nitrate, beta blocker, calcium channel blocker) may not be the best combination to treat this patient.

Chapter 28

1. sympathetic
2. alpha
3. alpha, beta

4. beta$_1$

5. basic life support

6. Whole blood

7. circulatory overload

8. PT, PTT, bleeding time

9. a   10. a   11. a   12. b   13. a   14. d

15. c   16. b   17. c   18. d   19. a   20. c

21. b   22. d   23. c   24. a   25. b   26. d

27. d   28. b   29. d   30. a   31. c

32. b

33. 13.86 mL/hr: 369.6 mcg/min

$$\frac{92.4 \text{ kg}}{1 \text{ min}} \times \frac{4 \text{ mcg}}{1 \text{ kg}} \times \frac{1 \text{ mg}}{1,000 \text{ mcg}} \times \frac{250 \text{ mL}}{400 \text{ mg}} \times \frac{60 \text{ min}}{1 \text{ h}}$$

$$= \frac{5,544,000}{400,000} = 13.86 \text{ mL/h}$$

$$\frac{400 \text{ mg}}{250 \text{ mL}} \times \frac{1,000 \text{ mcg}}{1 \text{ mg}} \times \frac{1 \text{ h}}{60 \text{ min}} \times \frac{13.86 \text{ mL}}{1 \text{ h}}$$

$$= \frac{5,544,000}{15,000} = \frac{369.60 \text{ mcg}}{\text{min}}$$

34. $$\frac{99.4 \text{ kg}}{1 \text{ min}} \times \frac{5 \text{ mcg}}{1 \text{ kg}} \times \frac{1 \text{ mg}}{1,000 \text{ mcg}} \times \frac{250 \text{ mL}}{500 \text{ mg}} \times \frac{60 \text{ min}}{1 \text{ h}}$$

$$= 14.91 \text{ mL/hr}$$

35. a. Assessment data include auto accident, wandering, confusion, weak pulse, dysrhythmia, changing blood pressure, pulse, and unresponsiveness.

b. *Altered Tissue Perfusion* (©2012 NANDA-I) related to changing pulse and blood pressure

c. Dextran is an IV colloid given to expand fluid volume. If blood pressure rises, the nurse can assume the drug is effective. Norepinephrine is a potent vasoconstrictor used to reverse the severe hypotension. If blood pressure rises, then the nurse knows the drug is effective. Dobutamine will help the heart beat with more force so that vital organs can receive blood and nutrients. When pulse becomes strong and blood pressure rises, the nurse can assume that the drug is effective. Lidocaine was given to correct the dysrhythmia. When heart rate and rhythm return to preaccident levels, then the nurse can assume the medication was effective.

36. a. With a closed head injury, neurogenic shock must be considered. The fact that the patient is comatose, has slow respirations, low blood pressure and pulse, and has unresponsive pupils supports this diagnosis.

b. Vasoconstrictors such as norepinephrine will likely be needed to maintain the patient's blood pressure; an inotropic drug such as dopamine may be useful in strengthening the force of the myocardial contraction.

c. Blood pressure, pulse, and respirations return to normal. The patient regains consciousness. No CPR is necessary and no tissue hypoxia results to the brain or kidney.

Chapter 29

1. sodium

2. supraventricular

3. sudden death

4. atrial fibrillation

5. sodium channels

6. slow, decrease

7. a. SA node

   b. AV node

   c. Bundle of His

   d. Bundle branches

   e. Purkinje fibers

   f. P wave

   g. QRS complex

   h. T wave

8. a   9. b   10. d   11. d   12. a   13. c

14. a   15. a   16. e   17. a   18. d   19. c

20. b   21. d   22. b   23. c   24. a   25. d

26. d   27. c   28. b   29. a   30. b   31. b

32. d   33. d   34. c   35. b   36. c   37. a

38. c   39. d   40. c   41. b

42. $$\frac{100 \text{ mL}}{125 \text{ mg}} \times \frac{20 \text{ mg}}{1 \text{ h}} = \frac{2,000}{125} = \frac{16 \text{ mL}}{\text{h}}$$

43. $$\frac{250 \text{ mL}}{900 \text{ mg}} \times \frac{0.5 \text{ mg}}{1 \text{ min}} \times \frac{60 \text{ min}}{1 \text{ h}} =$$

$$\frac{7,500}{900} = \frac{8.33 \text{ mL}}{\text{h}} \text{ or } \frac{8 \text{ mL}}{\text{h}}$$

44. a. Because propranolol decreases heart rate and slows conduction through the AV node, the nurse should document heart rate and rhythm before giving propranolol. The nurse should also assess for the presence of heart block, bradycardia, AV block, and asthma. A blood pressure assessment is essential before the delivery of propranolol.

b. Amiodarone is an antidysrhythmic drug, and is specifically given for serious ventricular tachycardia. It will prolong the refractory period.

c. Amiodarone can cause blurred vision, rashes, photosensitivity, nausea, vomiting, anorexia, fatigue, dizziness, and hypotension. It can also cause a serious pneumonia-like syndrome; therefore, the nurse should frequently assess pulmonary function. Common adverse effects of propranolol include hypotension and bradycardia. The nurse must be alert for the patient's complaints of dizziness and fatigue.

45. a. Assess cardiac rhythm. Do not give if patient is demonstrating heart block, severe hypotension, severe congestive failure, or cardiogenic shock. Make sure vital signs and ECG are documented before drug is given. Note shortness of breath, presence of cough, chest pain, and urinary output.

b. Teach the patient about heart rate and the need to notify the nurse if the rate goes below 60 beats/min. Watch for orthostatic hypotension, confusion, and chest pain. Do not give with grapefruit juice as it may increase the level of Calan. Hawthorne, an herbal supplement, can cause hypotension if given with Calan.

c. Nursing diagnoses include:

1. *Altered Tissue Perfusion* (©2012 NANDA-I) related to cardiac conduction abnormality

2. *Deficient Knowledge* (©2012 NANDA-I) related to medication regimen

3. *Risk for Injury* (©2012 NANDA-I) related to medication adverse effects

Chapter 30

1. A. prothrombin activator

   B. thrombin

   C. fibrinogen

2. plasmin

3. garlic

4. thrombolytics

5. Hemostatics

6. prothrombin time (PT), international normalized ratio (INR)

7. a	8. e	9. b	10. c	11. f	12. e
13. g	14. d	15. a	16. a	17. c	18. b
19. d	20. a	21. d	22. c	23. c	24. a
25. a	26. c	27. d	28. d	29. c	30. b
31. b	32. d	33. b	34. a	35. b	36. a
37. d	38. c				

39. $\dfrac{2{,}500 \text{ units}}{1 \text{ h}} \times \dfrac{1{,}000 \text{ mL}}{50{,}000 \text{ units}} - \dfrac{2{,}500{,}000}{50{,}000} = \dfrac{50 \text{ mL}}{h}$

40. $\dfrac{20{,}000 \text{ units}}{500 \text{ mL}} \times \dfrac{30 \text{ mL}}{1 \text{ h}} = \dfrac{1{,}200 \text{ units}}{h}$

$\dfrac{1{,}200 \text{ units}}{1 \text{ h}} \times \dfrac{24 \text{ h}}{1 \text{ day}} = \dfrac{28{,}800 \text{ units}}{day}$

41. a. The patient should use caution when engaged in activities that can cause bleeding, such as shaving, brushing teeth, trimming nails, and using kitchen knives. A soft toothbrush and an electric razor are safe choices. Contact activities, because of their high risk for injury, should be avoided.

b. The patient should report unusual bruising or bleeding such as nose bleeds, bleeding gums, black or red stools, heavy menstrual periods, or spitting up blood.

c. Aspirin or other medications containing salicylates should never be taken. Acetaminophen could be used for headaches. Feverfew, garlic, ginger, and arnica also should be avoided.

42. a. Alcohol abuse is a major irritant for GI ulcer formation. The chronic use of alcohol might contribute to ulceration. The use of warfarin also prolongs bleeding time; thus, the bright red blood during vomiting.

b. Nursing diagnoses are as follows:

1. *Altered Tissue Perfusion* (©2012 NANDA-I) related to blood loss (Outcome: The patient will experience a stable blood pressure and pulse. The patient will have no signs and symptoms of anoxia.)

2. *Deficient Knowledge* (©2012 NANDA-I) related to alcohol consumption (Outcome: The patient will demonstrate understanding of the long-term effects of alcohol consumption.)

3. *Deficient Knowledge* (©2012 NANDA-I) related to warfarin treatment (Outcome: The patient will demonstrate understanding of the drug's action by accurately describing drug side effects and precautions.)

c. Immediate IM administration of vitamin K could reverse the anticoagulation effects of warfarin. Administration of an hemostatic such as aminocaproic acid (Amicar), might reduce excessive bleeding from the ulcer site.

Chapter 31

1. erythropoiesis, erythropoietin

2. epoetin alfa (Epogen, Procrit)

3. platelets

4. leukocytes

5. Ferritin, hemosiderin

6. recycled

7. c	8. a	9. b	10. a	11. b	12. a
13. c	14. d	15. c	16. c	17. b	18. d
19. a	20. c	21. a	22. b	23. d	24. b
25. a	26. d	27. c	28. a	29. c	30. a
31. b					

32. $\dfrac{57 \text{ kg}}{1 \text{ day}} \times \dfrac{5 \text{ mcg}}{1 \text{ kg}} = \dfrac{285}{1} = \dfrac{285 \text{ mcg}}{day}$

33. No;

$\dfrac{66 \text{ lb}}{1 \text{ day}} \times \dfrac{1 \text{ kg}}{2.2 \text{ lb}} \times \dfrac{20 \text{ mcg}}{1 \text{ kg}} = \dfrac{1{,}320}{2.2} = \dfrac{600 \text{ mcg}}{day}$

34. a. Renal failure causes a decrease in the production of the hormone erythropoietin. This leads to decreased production of RBCs and anemia.

b. Hypertension is the most likely side effect. It is related to the increased hematocrit and also to the renal failure. Others include CVA, MI, and thrombophlebitis, all related to the increased hematocrit. It would be important to ask the patient if he had any blurred vision, slurred speech, transient weakness, chest pain, or calf pain during the nurse's assessment.

c. Topics to cover include the importance of keeping health care providers' appointments so that blood pressure can be monitored, how to self-administer SC injections, used needle disposal, reportable BP changes, and how to take his own blood pressure at home. Signs and symptoms of thrombophlebitis should be discussed. The patient should also be taught to maintain adequate dietary intake of iron, folate, and B_{12} and to maintain his renal diet.

35. a. He should tell the nurse that the cause of pernicious anemia is due to lack of the intrinsic factor, in this case probably caused by his chronic gastritis. Since oxygen is carried on the RBCs and he is anemic, the body cells are not getting adequate oxygen. This causes the tired, lethargic feeling.

    b. The patient should be told to inform other nurses that he uses vitamin B_{12}, particularly in view of its interaction with colchicine. The importance of monitoring potassium levels should be stressed. Instruction on self-administration may be needed. If the patient gives it parenterally, signs of anaphylaxis should be taught.

    c. An iron preparation would be used in cases of inadequate hemoglobin or inadequate RBCs. The problem in megaloblastic anemia is that the RBCs are not maturing properly. B_{12} will treat this problem.

36. a. Assessments include health history, allergies, history of bacterial or fungal infections, vital signs, and WBC with differential.

    b. The patient should be told that filgrastim may cause an elevation in liver enzymes. It may cause an allergic reaction. Because of the stimulation of bone marrow cells, it may produce bone pain.

    c. She needs to wash hands frequently; limit contact with crowds and people with colds; cook all foods; avoid fresh fruits, vegetables, and plants; limit exposure to children and animals; empty the bladder frequently; drink more water; and cough and deep breathe several times daily.

Chapter 32

1. humoral, antibodies
2. active
3. passive
4. cytokines
5. biologic response modifiers
6. superinfections
7. glucocorticoids (corticosteroids), antimetabolites, antibodies, calcineurin inhibitors

8. c	9. a	10. d	11. e	12. f	13. b
14. c	15. c	16. b	17. c	18. a	19. d
20. a	21. c	22. a	23. c	24. a	25. d
26. c	27. c	28. d	29. a	30. d	

31. 72 hours = 12,272.73 mg

$$\frac{180\ lb}{dose} \times \frac{1\ kg}{2.2\ lb} \times \frac{150\ mg}{1\ kg} = \frac{27,000}{2.2} = \frac{12,272.73}{dose}$$

2, 4, 6, 8 weeks = 8,181.82 mg

$$\frac{180\ lb}{dose} \times \frac{1\ kg}{2.2\ lb} \times \frac{100\ mg}{1\ kg} = \frac{18.00}{2.2} = \frac{8,181.82}{dose}$$

12 + 16 weeks = 4,090.91 mg

$$\frac{180\ lb}{dose} \times \frac{1\ kg}{2.2} \times \frac{50\ mg}{1\ kg} = \frac{9,000}{2.2} = \frac{4,090.91}{dose}$$

32. $$\frac{100\ lb}{dose} \times \frac{1\ kg}{2.2\ lb} \times \frac{0.15\ mg}{1\ kg} = \frac{15}{2.2} = \frac{6.82\ mg}{dose}$$

$$\frac{6.82\ mg}{dose} \times \frac{2\ dose}{1} = \frac{13.64\ mg}{24\ hours}$$

33. a. The immunostimulant therapy may cause a spontaneous abortion.

    b. Complications or adverse reactions include encephalopathy, depression, bone marrow depression, nausea, and stomatitis.

    c. Side effects include hematuria, petechiae, tarry stools, bruising, fever, sore throat, jaundice, dark-colored urine, clay-colored stools, feelings of sadness, and nervousness.

34. a. Immunosuppressants are used to dampen the immune response to reduce the possibility of transplant rejection. The patient may need to take the medication for the rest of her life.

    b. This class of drugs was developed to suppress the normal cell-mediated immune response. In lay terms, the medication the patient is taking keeps the patient's body from rejecting the new kidney.

    c. Adverse reactions include superimposed infections, bone marrow depression, alopecia, arthralgia, respiratory distress, edema, nausea, vomiting, paresthesia, fever, blood in urine, black stools, increased pigmentation, and feelings of sadness.

35. a. Vaccinations have eradicated smallpox and poliovirus. They have reduced diphtheria and measles to a fraction of their occurrence prior to vaccinations. They keep children healthy and reduce the chance for life-threatening diseases.

    b. The child may have a red area and a sore spot where the shot was given, but this is normal. Severe reactions are rare and usually occur at the time of the shot when help is readily available.

Chapter 33

1. contain the injury or destroy the microorganism
2. Mast
3. salicylism
4. nonsteroidal anti-inflammatory drugs (NSAIDs)
5. Corticosteroids (Glucocorticoids)
6. Cushing's
7. Reye's

8. c	9. a	10. a	11. c	12. b	13. d
14. c	15. a	16. a	17. d	18. c	19. a
20. c	21. d	22. b	23. b	24. d	25. b
26. d	27. a	28. c	29. c		

30. $$\frac{30\ \text{qtt}}{\text{dose}} \times \frac{1\ \text{mL}}{15\ \text{gtt}} = \frac{30}{15} = \frac{2\ \text{mL}}{\text{dose}}$$

$$\frac{2\ \text{mL}}{\text{dose}} \times \frac{6\ \text{doses}}{1} = \frac{12\ \text{mL}}{24\ \text{h}}$$

$$\frac{30\ \text{qtt}}{\text{dose}} \times \frac{6\ \text{doses}}{1} = \frac{180\ \text{qtt}}{24\ \text{h}}$$

31. $$\frac{500\ \text{mg}}{\text{dose}} \times \frac{1\ \text{tablet}}{250\ \text{mg}} = \frac{500}{250} = \frac{2\ \text{tablets}}{\text{dose}}$$

$$\frac{500\ \text{mg}}{\text{dose}} \times 4\ \text{dose} = \frac{2{,}000\ \text{mg}}{24\ \text{h}}$$

Not a recommended dose. 1,000 mg is recommended in a 24-hour period.

32. a. Empirin 2 in a combination drug of aspirin and codeine 2 mg. Aspirin is an anti-inflammatory/pain reliever and codeine is an opioid used for moderate pain. Ketoprofen is also an anti-inflammatory/pain reliever, but with greater anti-inflammatory properties than aspirin.

b. Corticosteroids are contraindicated when an active infection is present.

c. Aspirin is irritating to the stomach lining and with its anticoagulant effect may cause gastric bleeding. Codeine may cause constipation, nausea, and vomiting. Ketoprofen may also cause nausea and vomiting.

33. a. The drug classification is nonsteroidal anti-inflammatory drug (NSAID).

b. They have fewer GI side effects and do not affect blood coagulation.

c. The nurse should assess for heart failure (HF), fluid retention, hypertension, renal disease and liver dysfunction.

34. a. Children under the age of 19 years should not be given aspirin (ASA).

b. Children under 1 year of age should be given infant drops related to variations in the strengths in the preparations listed as "children's liquid."

c. Aspirin when given to children under the age of 19 may cause the potentially fatal condition Reye's syndrome.

Chapter 34

1. virulent
2. mutations
3. broad spectrum
4. superinfection
5. penicillinase (or beta-lactamase)
6. beta-lactamase inhibitor
7. Macrolide
8. aminoglycosides
9. a   10. f   11. b   12. e   13. e   14. d
15. c   16. b   17. g   18. f   19. a   20. b
21. f   22. b   23. e   24. c   25. a   26. c

27. c   28. d   29. b   30. c   31. d   32. c
33. d   34. d   35. d   36. b   37. b   38. b
39. a   40. d   41. a   42. a   43. c   44. b
45. d

46. $$\frac{500\ \text{mg}}{1} \times \frac{1\ \text{g}}{1000\ \text{mg}} = \frac{1\ \text{tablet}}{1\ \text{g}} = \frac{500}{1000} =$$

$$\frac{\frac{1}{2}\ \text{tablet}}{\text{dose}} = \frac{\frac{2}{1}\text{dose}}{1} = \frac{1\ \text{tablet}}{12\ \text{hr}}$$

47. $$\frac{500\ \text{mg}}{\text{dose}} \times \frac{1\ \text{tablet}}{250\ \text{mg}} = \frac{500}{250} = \frac{2\ \text{tablets}}{\text{dose}}$$

$$\frac{2\ \text{tablets}}{\text{dose}} \times \frac{4\ \text{dose}}{1} = \frac{8\ \text{tablets}}{24\ \text{hr}}$$

48. a. The widespread use of antibiotics often leads to resistant strains of bacteria.

b. The longer the antibiotic is used, the greater the percentage of resistant strains.

c. She may develop acquired resistance.

d. It will most likely become ineffective in treating her infection.

49. a. Broad-spectrum antibiotics are prescribed until the culture and sensitivity tests can be performed and the actual microbe can be identified.

b. Culture and sensitivity tests are performed to identify the microbe causing the infection.

c. Specific drug therapy can be selected based on which antibiotic would be most effective.

50. a. Adverse effects are formation of crystals in the urine, hypersensitivity reactions, nausea and vomiting, aplastic anemia, hemolytic anemia, and agranulocytosis.

b. The nurse must carefully monitor the patient's condition and provide patient education.

c. Encourage 3,000 mL fluid every 24 hours to reduce the possibility of the formation of crystals in the urine.

Chapter 35

1. Fungi
2. sporotrichosis, blastomycosis, histoplasmosis, coccidioidomycosis
3. candidiasis, aspergillosis, cryptococcosis, mucormycosis
4. mycoses
5. dermatophytic
6. lungs, brain, digestive organs
7. superficial, systemic
8. azoles, ergosterol
9. Amphotericin B
10. orally
11. a   12. b   13. a   14. a   15. b   16. a
17. c   18. a   19. d   20. b   21. e   22. f
23. d   24. d   25. c   26. c   27. a   28. a

29. d   30. b   31. a   32. c   33. a   34. b
35. c   36. a   37. b   38. a   39. a   40. d

41. $\dfrac{150\ lb}{1} \times \dfrac{1\ kg}{2.2\ lb} = \dfrac{150}{2.2} = 68.18\ kg$

$\dfrac{150\ lb}{day} \times \dfrac{1\ kg}{2.2\ lb} \times \dfrac{0.25\ mg}{1\ kg} = \dfrac{37.50}{2.2} = \dfrac{17.05\ mg}{day}$

42. 100 mg/50 mg × 1 = 2 tablets per dose

43. a. The patient should consult her obstetrician concerning the best choice for her drug regimen. Antifungals with fewer adverse reactions are more commonly used for vaginal candidiasis such as terconazole (Terazol) and tioconazole (Vagistat).

b. The foremost importance is to treat the problem without harming the fetus. Therefore, the drug of choice would be the antifungal with the least adverse reactions and the least potential for harm to the fetus.

44. a. The recommended drug regimen is chloroquine (Aralen) 600 mg initial dose and 300 mg weekly for acute attacks; primaquine for a total cure 15 mg every day for 2 weeks.

b. With low doses of chloroquine, nausea and diarrhea may be expected. Higher doses may lead to CNS and cardiovascular toxicity.

45. a. The patient will receive metronidazole (Flagyl) 250 to 750 mg tid.

b. Adverse reactions include anorexia, nausea, diarrhea, dizziness, headache, dryness of the mouth, and metallic taste in the mouth.

c. Amebiasis involves the large intestine and liver.

Chapter 36

1. capsid, ribonucleic acid (RNA), deoxyribonucleic acid (DNA)
2. intracellular parasites
3. latent
4. antiretroviral
5. highly active antiretroviral therapy
6. neuroaminidase inhibitors
7. protease inhibitors
8. DNA, contaminated blood, body fluids
9. Acyclovir
10. HCV
11. c   12. d   13. b   14. e   15. a   16. b
17. d   18. a   19. a   20. c   21. c   22. a
23. a   24. b   25. c   26. a   27. b   28. a
29. c   30. d   31. d

32. $\dfrac{100\ mg}{dose} \times \dfrac{1\ tablet}{50\ mg} = \dfrac{100}{50} = \dfrac{2\ tablets}{dose}$

$\dfrac{2\ tablets}{dose} \times \dfrac{2\ dose}{day} = \dfrac{4\ tablets}{day}$

33. $\dfrac{9\ mcg}{dose} \times \dfrac{1\ mL}{20\ mcg} = \dfrac{9}{20} = \dfrac{0.45\ mL}{dose}$

Use tubercular syringe.

34. a. The combination drug regimen is called highly active antiretroviral therapy (HAART). The goal of HAART is to reduce the plasma level of HIV to its lowest possible level; and to allow the patient to live symptom-free longer. HAART also reduces the probability that a virus will become resistant to treatment.

b. Classes include nucleoside reverse transcriptase inhibitors (NRTIs), nonnucleoside reverse transcriptase inhibitors (NNRTIs), protease inhibitors, entry inhibitors and integrase inhibitors.

c. NRTIs, prevent the viral DNA chain from lengthening. NNRTIs bind directly to the viral enzyme reverse transcriptase and inhibit its function. Protease inhibitors block the viral enzyme protease, which is responsible for the final assembly of the HIV virions. Fusion and integrase inhibitors block the ability of HIV to enter its host cell.

35. a. The vaccination may prevent the patient from getting influenza or reduce the severity of the symptoms.

b. The vaccination lasts several months to 1 year.

c. Amantadine (Symmetrel) is the drug of choice.

36. a. Transmission of HBV occurs through exposure to contaminated blood and body fluids.

b. Symptoms include fever, chills, fatigue, anorexia, nausea, and vomiting.

c. Symptoms include prolonged fatigue, jaundice, liver cirrhosis, and ultimately liver failure.

d. The current recommendation is universal vaccination of all children.

37. a. Cautious use of drug therapy is warranted during pregnancy.

b. Acyclovir (Zovirax) is the preferred drug.

c. Adverse effects are nephrotoxicity and hepatotoxicity.

Chapter 37

1. use of multiple drugs, special dosing schedules
2. alkylating agents
3. folic acid
4. intravenously
5. natural products
6. hormones, hormone
7. Biologic response
8. d   9. e   10. g   11. a   12. b   13. c
14. a   15. b   16. e   17. b   18. c   19. e
20. d   21. f   22. a   23. b   24. d   25. d
26. a   27. c   28. a   29. c   30. b   31. c
32. d   33. b   34. c   35. a   36. d   37. a
38. b   39. a   40. d   41. b
42. d

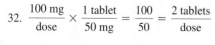

43. $\dfrac{20 \text{ mg}}{\text{dose}} \times \dfrac{1 \text{ tablet}}{10 \text{ mg}} = \dfrac{20}{10} = \dfrac{2 \text{ tablets}}{\text{dose}}$

44. $\dfrac{25 \text{ mg}}{\text{dose}} \times \dfrac{2 \text{ mL}}{50 \text{ mg}} = \dfrac{50}{50} = \dfrac{1 \text{ mL}}{\text{dose}}$

$\dfrac{1 \text{ mL}}{\text{dose}} \times \dfrac{4 \text{ dose}}{1} = \dfrac{4 \text{ mL}}{\text{day}}$

45. a. Tumors should be treated at an early age with multiple drugs and using several methods such as chemotherapy, radiation, and surgery when possible. If the patient had not sought medical treatment early enough, the remaining cancer cells could decrease the chance of recovery.

b. Drugs from different antineoplastic classes can be given during a course of chemotherapy. Different classes might affect different stages of the cancer cell's life cycle, thereby increasing the percentage of cancer cell death.

c. Administer drugs on a specific schedule to give normal cells time to recover from the adverse effects of the drugs.

46. a. Medications include antiemetics, benzodiazepines, serotonin receptor antagonists, and corticosteroids.

b. The patient should avoid crowds, unsanitary conditions, and other potentially infectious situations. Proper hygiene is strongly recommended.

c. Anorexia can be reduced by providing the patient with her favorite foods. A well-balanced diet should be implemented, including consultation with a registered dietician.

47. a. Tamoxifen causes initial "tumor flare," an idiosyncratic increase in tumor size and bone, but this is an expected therapeutic event.

b. Tamoxifen is a selective estrogen receptor modulator (SERM).

c. The drug is effective against breast tumors that require estrogen for their growth.

d. Tamoxifen is one of the few antineoplastics given to *prevent* cancer, as well as to *treat* cancer.

e. No, this medication is a pregnancy category D and has been determined to have adverse effects on the fetus. It should be given only if the benefits to the mother outweigh the risks to the fetus.

Chapter 38

1. mucous membranes
2. antihistamines, intranasal corticosteroids, mast cell stabilizers
3. antihistamines
4. sympathomimetics
5. dextromethorphan

6. a	7. b	8. c	9. a	10. b	11. c
12. b	13. a	14. c	15. b	16. d	17. b
18. c	19. a	20. d	21. a	22. a	23. c

24. c	25. c	26. a	27. b	28. a	29. d
30. a	31. d	32. c	33. a	34. b	35. d

36. 150 mg

37. 12 mL

38. a. *Deficient Knowledge* (©2012 NANDA-I) related to medication change evidenced by patient asking questions

b. Assess patient knowledge of the medications that she has been taking and of her condition.

c. Teach patient about side effects of the medications, reason for administration, and when to take them.

Write instructions for patient to take home. Answer specific questions by the patient:

1. Reasons for administration:
   a. Antibiotics are for infection in ear and lung. Take antibiotics as ordered until prescription runs out.
2. Proventil Inhaler:
   a. Take only every 4 hours as prescribed.
   b. Be sure patient knows appropriate manner to set up the inhalation device.
   c. Proventil decreases wheezing and can be used to increase respiratory effectiveness.
   d. Proventil only needs to be used until symptoms improve.
3. Tylenol:
   a. Take for fever or pain, no more than 1 g every 4 h as needed.
4. Robitussin AC:
   a. Guaifenesin with codeine: Guaifenesin is an expectorant. Patient should consume at least 3 L of fluid per day. Codeine is a narcotic cough suppressant. Codeine causes drowsiness and itching. Robitussin is used to thin and remove secretions. Do not drive while taking codeine.
5. Sudafed:
   a. Sudafed is a decongestant used to decrease stuffy nose and fluid in the ear. It may cause insomnia. Take only as directed on package.
6. Benadryl:
   a. It is not recommended because of its drying effect on mucous membranes in the lung.
   b. Notify the health care provider or return to clinic if condition worsens or there is no improvement.

Chapter 39

1. perfusion, ventilation
2. nebulizer
3. emphysema, chronic bronchitis
4. respiration
5. 12 to 18; emotion, fever, stress, pH
6. constriction
7. metered dose inhaler (MDI)
8. Status asthmaticus
9. terminate, frequency

10. e   11. a   12. f   13. g   14. e   15. b
16. d   17. c   18. e   19. d   20. c   21. b
22. d   23. a   24. b   25. c   26. b   27. d
28. a   29. b   30. c   31. c   32. a   33. a
34. d   35. c   36. b   37. a   38. c

39. $\dfrac{50\ \text{kg}}{1\ \text{h}} \times \dfrac{0.25\ \text{mg}}{1\ \text{kg}} = \dfrac{12.50\ \text{kg}}{1\ \text{h}} * \dfrac{6\ \text{h}}{1} = 75\ \text{mg}$

40. $\dfrac{4\ \text{mg}}{\text{dose}} \times \dfrac{5\ \text{mL}}{2\ \text{mg}} = \dfrac{20}{2} = \dfrac{10\ \text{mL}}{\text{dose}}$

41. a. Assessment: Green, thick mucus. Increased incidence of wheezing and shortness of breath and wheezing worsening over 2 weeks.

  b. Interventions are as follows:

   1. Assess respiratory status, respiratory rate, vital signs, auscultation of breath sounds, pulmonary function studies; peak flow, ABGs, and O_2 saturations.

   2. Administer fluids: IV if necessary, PO if possible: 2–3 L per day

   3. Elevant the head of the bed.

   4. Administer O_2 as needed to maintain oxygen levels in satisfactory level.

   5. Administer beta$_2$ agonist and monitor for improvement and adverse effects.

   6. Patient teaching to include:

    a. Preventive inhaler (beclomethasone)

    b. Fluids: 3 L per day

    c. Notify the health care provider for any increased dyspnea, wheezing, fever, change in sputum color or consistency.

    d. Encourage compliance with medications and discuss side effects and ways to decrease adverse effects.

    e. Avoid environmental antigens that trigger asthma responses such as pollen, animal dander, dust, smoke, and cold air.

    f. Eat regularly using smaller meals more frequently.

    g. Receive yearly vaccines to prevent respiratory infections.

    h. Decrease or eliminate intake of caffeine.

    i. Avoid smoking.

  c. Beclomethasone is a corticosteroid used to decrease inflammation and prevent asthma attacks. Theophylline is a xanthine bronchodilator used to provide bronchodilation.

  d. Ativan is a CNS depressant that is used as an antianxiety agent to decrease the dyspnea due to stress and anxiety. Metaproterenol is a beta$_2$ agonist that will dilate the bronchi and relieve the dyspnea.

Chapter 40

1. alimentary, accessory
2. transport, enzymes, digestion, absorption

3. villi, microvilli, medications
4. peristalsis, smooth
5. cardiac sphincter, esophageal reflux
6. chief, parietal, intrinsic factor
7. acidic, 1.5 to 3.5
8. glucocorticoids, aspirin, NSAIDs
9. *Helicobacter pylori*
10. e   11. c   12. a   13. f   14. d   15. b
16. a   17. b   18. d   19. d   20. a   21. d
22. c   23. b   24. d   25. c   26. d   27. b
28. b   29. d   30. c   31. b   32. a

33. a. $\dfrac{60\ \text{gtt}}{1\ \text{mL}} \times \dfrac{100\ \text{mL}}{30\ \text{min}} \times \dfrac{60\ \text{min}}{1\ \text{h}} = \dfrac{360,000}{30} =$
   $\dfrac{360,000}{30} = \dfrac{12,000\ \text{qtts}}{\text{h}}$

  b. $\dfrac{100\ \text{mL}}{30\ \text{min}} \times \dfrac{60\ \text{min}}{1\ \text{h}} = \dfrac{6000}{30} = \dfrac{200\ \text{mL}}{\text{h}}$

34. a. 1,000, 1,400, 1,900, 2,200 hours

  b. $\dfrac{2\ \text{T}}{1} \times \dfrac{3\ \text{tsp}}{1\ \text{T}} = 6\ \text{tsp}$
   $\dfrac{2\ \text{T}}{1} \times \dfrac{15\ \text{mL}}{1\ \text{T}} = 30\ \text{mL}$
   $\dfrac{2\ \text{T}}{1} \times \dfrac{1\ \text{oz}}{2\ \text{T}} = \dfrac{2}{2} = 1\ \text{oz}$

35. a. Nursing diagnoses include *Risk for Injury* (©2012 NANDA-I) and *Deficient Knowledge* (©2012 NANDA-I).

  b. *Risk for Injury* (©2012 NANDA-I) is the priority diagnosis due to existing confusion. *Deficient Knowledge* (©2012 NANDA-I) is related to OTC medication to prevent further confusion.

36. a. The short-term goal is that the patient will be free from injury and will exhibit less confusion.

  b. Liver function tests need to be monitored, as cimetidine and ranitidine can be hepatotoxic.

37. a. The nursing diagnosis is *Deficient Knowledge* (©2012 NANDA-I) due to new medications.

  b. Do not take OTC meds before checking with the nurse due to drug–drug interactions.

  c. Antacids should be given 2 hours before or 2 hours after other medications because of drug–drug interactions and the effect of antacids on the gastric pH.

Chapter 41

1. stress; sights, sounds, smells
2. anticholinergics, antihistamines
3. emetics, ipecac, vomiting
4. Anorexiants, moderate
5. frequency, bowel movements
6. food intake, dietary fiber
7. impaction, obstruction

Adams/Holland, *Student Workbook and Resource Guide for Pharmacology for Nurses* 4th Edition
© 2014 by Pearson Education, Inc.

8. laxative, defecation

9. monitoring, education

10. esophageal obstruction, intestinal obstruction, fecal impaction

11. b	12. g	13. e	14. a	15. d	16. f
17. c	18. c	19. c	20. a	21. d	22. c
23. a	24. a	25. d	26. c	27. b	28. a
29. c	30. b	31. c	32. c	33. a	34. c

35. a. $\dfrac{10 \text{ mg}}{\text{dose}} \times \dfrac{2 \text{ mL}}{25 \text{ mg}} = \dfrac{20}{25} = \dfrac{0.8 \text{ mL}}{\text{dose}}$

b. 3-mL syringe

c. For average size adult, 20–21 gauge, 1–1 1/2 inch needle

36. $\dfrac{2.5 \text{ mg}}{\text{dose}} \times \dfrac{4 \text{ dose}}{\text{day}} = \dfrac{10 \text{ mg}}{\text{day}}$

37. a. *Risk for Injury* (©2012 NANDA-I) and *Deficient Knowledge* (©2012 NANDA-I) are two important nursing diagnoses for this patient.

b. The patient will be free from physical injury related to frequency of stools and physical weakness. The patient will understand the signs and symptoms of complications and report them appropriately.

c. Nursing actions include providing a clutter-free environment with a commode at the bedside and a call bell within reach, and monitoring for stools (amount and character).

d. Criteria include abdominal assessment for presence of bowel sounds, palpation for softness of and pain-free abdomen, and the act of defecation.

38. a. The initial assessment will include vital signs, evidence of weakness or confusion, and abdominal assessment.

b. Objective data include vital signs, abdominal assessment, number of stools visualized with color, and character of stool.

c. Safety issues are ensuring that the call bell is within reach; the ability to follow directions and call for help; the commode is at the bedside; the environment is clutter free; and slippers are available.

39. a. The initial assessment will include vital signs, adequate nutrition, absence of vomiting, stable laboratory studies, and lack of uterine contractions.

b. The primary goal is a full-term pregnancy without harm to fetus or mother.

c. Compazine is a pregnancy category C, so the risks must be weighed as fetal harm in animals has been noted.

d. Outcome criteria will include (1) vital signs and weight (no further loss of weight); (2) laboratory results (stable electrolytes), Hgb, and Hct; and (3) intake and output (adequate nutrition and hydration).

40. a. A low-fat diet should be maintained while on Xenical and fat-soluble vitamin supplements should be added to the diet.

b. Supplemental multivitamins with D, E, K, and beta carotene should be taken daily; psyllium may be taken at bed time to decrease GI side effects.

c. Provide psychological support and patient education reinforcing the difference between hunger and appetite accompanied by diversional therapy. A nutritional consult is needed to assess for healthy foods among what the patient likes.

Chapter 42

1. organic compounds, growth, normal metabolic processes

2. D, synthesize

3. prothrombin, blood clotting

4. lipid soluble; A, D, E, and K

5. Fat-soluble, small intestine, liver

6. Dietary Allowance (RDA), minimum, deficiency

7. Hypervitaminosis; A, C, D, E, B_6, niacin, and folic acid

8. Alcohol abuse

9. ergocalciferol

10. Vitamin E, free radicals, membranes

11. e	12. d	13. a	14. b	15. g	16. c
17. f	18. d	19. a	20. d	21. a	22. a
23. c	24. b	25. a	26. d	27. a	28. a
29. a	30. a	31. c	32. c		

33. $\dfrac{200 \text{ mcg}}{\text{mo}} \times \dfrac{\text{mL}}{100 \text{ mcg}} = \dfrac{200}{100} = \dfrac{2 \text{ mL}}{\text{mo}}$

34. $\dfrac{250 \text{ mL}}{4 \text{ h}} = \dfrac{62.50 \text{ mL}}{\text{h}}$

35. a. Pulmocare is specialized for respiratory patients.

b. Protein and albumin levels will need to be monitored as well as electrolytes, glucose, and kidney function tests.

c. The four types of enteral feedings are oligomeric, polymeric, modular, and specialized.

d. The overall goal for this patient is to have his nutritional status meet body requirements.

e. Nursing interventions include monitoring daily weights, intake and output, and lab values to determine the success of the plan.

f. Evaluative criteria will include (1) respiratory assessment (especially right middle lobe to note clearing or absence of adventitious sounds); and (2) daily weights with maintenance of body weight and adequate intake and output.

36. a. The patient will receive hyperalimentation with high caloric intake, supplemented by vitamins and trace minerals.

b. The TPN is indicated for impaired swallowing poststroke. A central line is necessary for TPN longer than 2 weeks to avoid phlebitis in peripheral veins secondary to the delivery of a hyperosmolar solution administered intravenously.

c. The short-term goal is that the patient will be free from hyper- and hypoglycemic reactions.

d. The long-term goal is that the patient will receive adequate nutrition allowing for a change to enteral feedings.

e. The nurse will monitor for the following:

　1. Hyper/hypoglycemic reactions and blood glucose

　2. Respiratory status and vital signs

　3. Insertion site for signs of infection

　4. Daily weight and intake and output

f. Patient will not experience difficulty breathing, will remain infection free, and will maintain moderate weight gain.

37. a. For long-term therapy, peripheral veins are not sufficient because of phlebitis. A NANDA diagnosis is *Nutrition, More than Body Requires* (©2012 NANDA-I).

b. This type of feeding will be necessary for 6 weeks or more; patient will be infection free and maintain stable lab results.

c. The patient can go home with home care support in the community.

Chapter 43

1. Hormones

2. fluid, electrolyte

3. desmopressin (DDAVP), vasopressin

4. cardiovascular

5. anxiety

6. with

7. infection

8. c	9. d	10. e	11. a	12. b	13. c
14. a	15. b	16. d	17. d	18. c	19. b
20. a	21. a	22. b	23. d	24. c	25. b
26. d	27. a	28. a	29. b	30. c	31. b
32. a	33. d	34. c			

35. $\dfrac{10 \text{ units}}{\text{dose}} \times \dfrac{1 \text{ mL}}{2 \text{ units}} = \dfrac{10}{20} = \dfrac{0.5 \text{ mL}}{\text{dose}}$

36. $\dfrac{200 \text{ mg}}{\text{dose}} \times \dfrac{204 \text{ tablet}}{50 \text{ mg}} = \dfrac{200}{50} = \dfrac{4 \text{ tablets}}{\text{dose}}$

37. a. Thyroid preparations increase metabolic activity. They may elevate body temperature, increase heart rate, and reduce the patient's weight. The effects of thyroid medications increase when a patient is also taking insulin.

b. The nurse should take a thorough health history, communicate findings with the prescribing health care provider, and teach the patient to report adverse effects promptly.

38. a. PTU may cause vital sign changes. The patient should be taught how to monitor his or her vital signs and to report changes promptly. This may require the purchase of necessary equipment. Risk of infection increases with the use of PTU. The patient must understand the importance of avoiding crowds

and individuals with known illnesses. This may lead to feelings of isolation.

b. The nurse can assist by encouraging alternative methods of communication such as the telephone and computer when susceptibility is increased. Because drowsiness may occur with the use of this medication, teaching concerning safety is of importance. The nurse should instruct the patient to avoid being near environmental hazards, driving, and operating machinery.

Chapter 44

1. type 1 diabetes mellitus, type 2 diabetes mellitus

2. oral hypoglycemics

3. resistant

4. blood glucose

5. a	6. b	7. b	8. d	9. c	10. b
11. a	12. e	13. a	14. c	15. c	16. d
17. d	18. d	19. b	20. a	21. b	22. c
23. c	24. b	25. a	26. b		
27. a					

28. 35 units + 20 units = 55 units

29. $\dfrac{10 \text{ mg}}{\text{dose}} \times \dfrac{1 \text{ tablet}}{5 \text{ mg}} = \dfrac{10}{5} = \dfrac{2 \text{ tablets}}{\text{dose}}$

30. a. Pharmacotherapy for type 2 diabetes is usually oral hypoglycemic agents, and lifestyle changes such as proper diet and increased level of activity will be necessary.

b. Because the patient is elderly, these approaches may be a problem as older patients are not as active as the general population, and they do not easily comply with instructions for a change of diet. Additionally, if the patient has other physical limitations because of his age or if he is not able to receive proper instruction because of these limitations (seeing or hearing, for example), these could be obstacles to diabetic therapy.

31. a. The following are hypoglycemic signs observed in patients with either type 1 diabetes or type 2 diabetes:

　1. Polyuria—excessive urination

　2. Polyphagia—increase in hunger

　3. Polydipsia—increased thirst

　4. Glucosuria—high levels of glucose in the urine

　5. Change in weight

　6. Fatigue

b. Initially, the following general areas should be monitored and reviewed:

　1. Obtain a complete health history including allergies, drug history, and possible drug interactions.

　2. Review lab tests for any abnormalities.

　3. Obtain an accurate history of alcohol use.

　4. Monitor blood glucose.

5. Monitor for signs and symptoms of illness or infection.

6. Monitor weight, weighing at the same time of day each time. This should be done for a time necessary to determine a pattern of weight loss or weight gain.

7. Monitor activity level.

8. Assess appetite and presence of symptoms that indicate patient may not be able to consume or retain the next meal.

9. Monitor blood pressure and other vital signs.

10. Assess lifestyle habits that might affect patient's physical condition and approaches for pharmacotherapy (smoking, eating patterns, substance misuse or abuse).

c. Patient education as it relates to oral hypoglycemic drugs would include goals for pharmacotherapy, importance of diet and exercise, reasons for obtaining baseline data such as vital signs and cardiac and renal function tests, and recognizing symptoms of hypoglycemia. Once a specific approach for pharmacotherapy has been determined, the following are additional points the nurse should include when teaching patients:

1. Always carry a source of simple sugar in case of hypoglycemic reactions.

2. Wear a medic alert bracelet to alert emergency personnel of the diabetes.

3. Notify caregivers, coworkers, and others who may be able to render assistance.

4. Avoid the use of alcohol to avoid an Antabuse-like reaction.

5. Maintain specified diet and exercise regimen while on antidiabetic drugs, as these activities will help to keep blood glucose within a normal range.

6. Swallow tablets whole and do not crush sustained-release tablets.

7. Take medication 30 minutes before breakfast, or as directed by the health care provider.

Chapter 45

1. Follicle-stimulating hormone, luteinizing hormone
2. menopause
3. amenorrhea
4. progestins
5. prolactin, oxytocin
6. d   7. c   8. b   9. a   10. b   11. c
12. a   13. e   14. d   15. d   16. d   17. d
18. b   19. b   20. a   21. c   22. a   23. c
24. c   25. c   26. c   27. d   28. b   29. a
30. b   31. c

32. $\dfrac{100 \text{ mL}}{2 \text{ h}} \times \dfrac{15 \text{ gtt}}{1 \text{ mL}} \times \dfrac{1 \text{ h}}{60 \text{ min}} = \dfrac{1500}{120} =$

$\dfrac{12.50 \text{ qtt}}{\text{min}} = \dfrac{13 \text{ qtt}}{\text{min}}$

33. $\dfrac{100 \text{ mg}}{\text{dose}} \times \dfrac{1 \text{ mL}}{400 \text{ mq}} = \dfrac{100}{400} = \dfrac{0.25 \text{ mL}}{\text{dose}}$

34. a. The patient has a knowledge deficit related to the prescribed drug regimen. The desired outcome is for the patient to understand the drug regimen and manage her regimen appropriately.

b. Estrogen replacement therapy may be prescribed short term to alleviate unpleasant symptoms occurring during and after menopause. Hot flashes, night sweats, vaginal dryness, susceptibility to infection, erratic menstrual cycle, and nervousness may be reduced. The short-term risks of estrogen replacement therapy are bloating, nausea, vaginal bleeding, breast tenderness, and other common menstrual symptoms. The long-term risks of estrogen replacement therapy are ovarian cancer, gallbladder disease, and breast cancer.

35. a. The nurse must use this medication with caution and continuously monitor maternal and fetus status. Adverse effects of oxytocin include fetal dysrhythmias, neonatal jaundice, and intracranial hemorrhage related to possible fetal trauma. Maternal effects include cardiac arrhythmias, hypertensive episodes, water intoxication, uterine rupture or uterine hypotonicity, seizures, postpartum hemorrhage, and coma.

b. Changes in maternal and fetal vital signs must be reported immediately and the infusion stopped. Intake and output should be monitored closely. Contraction status during labor and fundal checks in the postpartum period are of utmost importance. The nurse must understand that uterine hypotonicity in the postpartum period is related to postpartum hemorrhage.

Chapter 46

1. Anabolic steroids
2. virilization (masculinization)
3. sildenafil (Viagra)
4. Benign prostatic hyperplasia (BPH)
5. Androgens
6. X   7. a   8. b   9. c   10. a   11. b
12. b   13. d   14. a   15. a   16. b   17. c
18. d   19. c   20. a   21. a   22. d   23. b
24. c   25. d   26. a   27. b

28. $\dfrac{150 \text{ mg}}{\text{dose}} \times \dfrac{1 \text{ tablet}}{100 \text{ mg}} = \dfrac{150}{100} = \dfrac{1.5 \text{ tablets}}{\text{dose}}$

29. $\dfrac{4 \text{ mg}}{\text{dose}} \times \dfrac{1 \text{ capsule}}{2 \text{ mg}} = \dfrac{4}{2} = \dfrac{2 \text{ capsules}}{\text{dose}}$

30. a. The nurse should teach the patient that the goal of finasteride (Proscar) therapy is to reduce urinary

symptoms related to an enlarged prostate. Urinary symptoms such as hesitancy, difficulty starting the stream, decreased diameter of the stream, nocturia, dribbling, and frequency should be diminished. The nurse should explain to the patient that it may be necessary to take Proscar for the remainder of his life to keep the symptoms under control.

b. To evaluate effectiveness of therapy, the nurse should devise a method of follow-up to assess the resolution of urinary symptoms. The patient should also be encouraged to contact his nurse if symptoms worsen.

31. a. The nurse should obtain a list of herbs used by the patient. If he uses echinacea in conjunction with androgen therapy, his insulin requirements may decrease, necessitating a change in his insulin dosage.

b. The patient should be instructed to carefully monitor his blood glucose during androgen therapy and be encouraged to report symptoms of hypoglycemia such as sweating, tremors, anxiety, or vertigo.

Chapter 47

1. Metabolic bone disease (MBD)
2. parathyroid, thyroid
3. vitamin D
4. rickets
5. osteoporosis, Paget's disease
6. parathyroid hormone, calcitonin
7. calcifediol, calcitriol
8. complexed, elemental
9. bisphosphonates, calcitonin
10. Disease-modifying antirheumatic drugs (DMARDs)
11. uricosurics
12. b   13. a   14. e   15. c   16. d   17. e
18. c   19. c   20. a   21. b   22. d   23. e
24. c   25. b   26. d   27. d   28. a   29. c
30. b   31. b   32. d   33. b   34. c   35. a
36. d   37. c   38. a   39. d   40. c   41. b
42. a

43. $\dfrac{4 \text{ mg}}{\text{maximum dose}} \times \dfrac{1 \text{ tablet}}{0.5 \text{ mg}} = \dfrac{4}{0.5} = \dfrac{8 \text{ tablets}}{\text{maximum dose}}$

44. $\dfrac{400 \text{ mg}}{\text{dose}} \times \dfrac{1 \text{ tablet}}{200 \text{ mg}} = \dfrac{400}{200} = \dfrac{2 \text{ tablets}}{\text{dose}}$

45. a. The symptoms the patient is experiencing are normal for his condition. Allopurinol (Lopurin) is used for gout flare-up and primary and secondary hyperuricemia.

b. To allay the pain, NSAIDs would probably be administered with antigout therapy. Medications could be administered with meals to minimize gastric upset.

Other expected effects would include diarrhea and rash. Precautions would be taken to minimize these symptoms. Over a longer time, difficulty in urination may occur.

c. During drug therapy, laboratory tests (BUN and creatinine) would be ordered to monitor whether the kidneys are functioning properly. Fluid intake and output would be monitored. Because allopurinol may cause bone-marrow depression, blood cell counts would be taken regularly. Liver function tests would also be ordered.

46. a. Patients with kidney disease are unable to synthesize the active form of vitamin D from the precursors formed by the body or taken in the diet. Calcium is not absorbed well from the GI tract unless there is adequate vitamin D, so the patient may become hypocalcemic.

b. The patient should be informed that periodic liver function tests will be necessary, as well as calcium, magnesium, and phosphate levels. The drug should be taken exactly as directed so that toxic levels do not develop. Fatigue, weakness, nausea, and vomiting should be reported. Alcohol and other liver-toxic drugs should be avoided. Exposure to 20 minutes of sunlight daily will help increase the amount of vitamin D available to the patient.

c. Again, the importance of routine lab studies for calcium levels must be stressed. Oral calcium supplements should be taken with meals or within an hour after meals. The patient should be advised to consume calcium-rich foods such as dark green, leafy vegetables and dairy products.

47. a. Osteoporosis occurs when the rate of bone replacement is less than the rate of bone breakdown. People at risk for osteoporosis include postmenopausal women, those who use excess alcohol or caffeine, those with anorexia nervosa, smokers, inactive persons, those who lack adequate vitamin D or calcium in their diets, and persons using corticosteroids, antiseizure medications, and immunosuppressive drugs. The disease can be detected through the use of bone density tests.

b. Medications used to treat osteoporosis include calcium and vitamin D therapy, estrogen replacement therapy, estrogen receptor modulators, bisphosphonates, and calcitonin.

c. The patient will need to be instructed that alendronate (Fosamax) decreases the breakdown of her bones. The usual side effects are GI problems such as nausea, vomiting, abdominal pain, and esophageal irritation. The drug should be taken on an empty stomach once a week. To prevent the esophagus from becoming irritated, the patient should not lie down for 30 minutes after taking the medication. Patient teaching for raloxifene (Evista) should include the need for periodic bone density scans. Sudden chest pain, dyspnea, pain in calves, and swelling in the legs should be reported promptly. The patient should not take estrogen replacement therapy while using this drug. In addition, safety measures regarding falls should be discussed, as well as the need for weight-bearing activity and adequate dietary consumption of calcium and vitamin D.

Chapter 48

1. keratolytic
2. scabies
3. retinoids
4. Psoralens
5. pruritus
6. antibiotics, oral contraceptives
7. eczema

8. c	9. d	10. e	11. c	12. a	13. b
14. c	15. d	16. c	17. e	18. a	19. b
20. c	21. b	22. a	23. d	24. d	25. d
26. c	27. b	28. b	29. d	30. a	31. b
32. b	33. b	34. c	35. d	36. c	

37. a. Because lindane has the potential to cause serious nervous system toxicity, it is now prescribed only after other less toxic drugs have failed to produce a therapeutic response. Lindane should be used cautiously in children under 10 years of age, and only if other pediculicides fail. Since this is the case here, the mother needs to know that lindane might cause local skin irritation and adverse CNS effects such as restlessness, dizziness, tremors, or convulsions. This usually occurs after misuse or ingestion. This shampoo must be kept out of the reach of smaller children in the household. It should not be applied to open skin lesions or used if the child has seizures. The mother should wear gloves while applying the shampoo, particularly if she is pregnant. The shampoo should remain on the hair for at least 5 minutes. Using tepid water will decrease itching.

b. The child's school nurse or teacher should be notified, as well as the parents of the child with whom she spent the night, and any other children who attended the sleepover. Anyone else with whom the child has had close contact (grandparents, for example) should be notified as well.

c. Children in school should not swap clothing or towels. Coat and hat racks at school may need to be eliminated to prevent the spread from one child to another. Combs or other hygiene supplies should not be shared, and bodily contact with an infected person should be avoided. Also, the child should not sleep with brothers or sisters until the problem is resolved. The nurse should stress that this is not a problem of social class, but simply an event that occurs when there is close contact.

38. a. The nurse would ask the patient if he has had nausea, vomiting, chills, and headache, as well as assessing the amount of pain and extent of the erythema. Also ask about sunburn and tanning history, the amount of time the patient usually spends in the sun before beginning to burn, and if he uses sunscreen products. An allergy history is also necessary.

b. Soothing lotions, rest, prevention of dehydration, and topical anesthetic agents may help. The topical anesthetics may be chilled prior to application to increase the cooling effect. In severe cases, aspirin or ibuprofen may be used.

c. Medication should not be applied to broken skin. If this occurs, call the health care provider. Prevent sunburn by decreasing exposure to sunlight, or by increasing the SPF number of the sunscreen. Wear a broad-brimmed hat, UV protection for the eyes, and a long-sleeved shirt if extended exposure to sunlight is expected during peak hours of the day. Sunburn results from overexposure to UV light and is associated with light skin complexions. Chronic sun exposure can lead to eye injury, cataracts, and skin cancer.

39. a. The causes of acne are unknown, although some factors associated with it have been identified. Overproduction of sebum by oil glands, keratin that blocks oil glands, and certain bacteria grow within oil gland openings and change the sebum to an irritating substance. This results in small, inflamed bumps on the skin. Other factors include the male hormone, which regulates the activity of the sebaceous glands.

b. A mental health history should be taken to determine whether the patient has had a history of depression or suicidal tendencies. Patients with seizures who use carbamazepine should be identified, because there is an increased risk for seizures. Also, oral antidiabetic agents may not be as effective, so the nurse should assess for diabetes, heart disease, and elevated lipid levels. Before the drug is used, a patch test must be done to test for sensitivity.

c. He should be told to monitor foods and avoid those that seem to make his acne worse. He can be taught to keep a food log to help determine which ones these are. Products that will irritate the skin, such as cologne, perfumes, and other alcohol-based products, should be avoided. If severe inflammation occurs during therapy, the health care provider should be notified. Use of OTC agents should be avoided unless approved by the provider.

Chapter 49

1. blockage, outflow, excessive production
2. open-angle glaucoma
3. miotics
4. mydriatics
5. cycloplegics
6. external otitis
7. otitis media
8. mastoiditis

9. a	10. b	11. b	12. b	13. a	14. a
15. a	16. f	17. g	18. b	19. d	20. c

21. d   22. e   23. b   24. b   25. b   26. a
27. c   28. d   29. d   30. c   31. a   32. b
33. a   34. c   35. a   36. c   37. d   38. b
39. b   40. a   41. a   42. a

43. $\dfrac{250 \text{ mg}}{24 \text{ h dose}} \times \dfrac{3 \text{ doses}}{1} = \dfrac{750 \text{ mg}}{24 \text{ h}}$

44. No need to verify the order—this is the standard way to administer pilocarpine in an emergency situation. (Of course, if the nurse is unsure of anything, it is always best to check it out before moving ahead!)

45. a. There is no permanent cure for glaucoma. Medications will have to be used indefinitely. Several classes of eye medications may be used alone or in combination to control the intraocular pressure problem characteristic of glaucoma.

    b. Xalatan is used to decrease the IOP. Side effects may include conjunctival edema, tearing, dryness, burning, pain, itching, photophobia, or visual disturbances. The eyelashes on the treated eye may grow, thicken, and darken. The iris may have color changes, as well as the skin around the eye. Generalized flulike symptoms may occur. The patient should remove contacts prior to administering and leave them out for 15 minutes. Wait 5 minutes between different eye medications.

    c. The patient should be instructed to report any visual changes, and any changes in medications or new health-related problems. He should be taught the proper way to administer eye drops and told to schedule them around his daily routines. Signs of side effects should be reported. He will need to know that measurements of intraocular pressure will be done periodically. For his safety, environmental lighting needs to be adjusted when dark and may need to be dimmed if there is photophobia.

    d. Intraocular pressure should be measured using tonometry at regular intervals to determine the effectiveness of the medication.

46. a. Additional assessments needed include the patient's allergy history and whether his mother knows how to administer the drugs properly and is aware of potential side effects.

    b. The patient's mother needs teaching regarding the correct use of ear drops and the fact that aspirin is contraindicated in young children because of the risk of Reye's syndrome. Teaching should include the following: Ear drops are contraindicated in cases where the eardrum has perforated. This is the most likely cause of the drainage in the patient's ear and may be seen on examination of the tympanic membrane. Explain that the bacteria present in the outer ear may be carried into the middle ear when the drops run in, thus increasing the chances of a further infection. The patient's mother needs to be made aware that ear drops should be warmed by holding under warm water prior to administration. Also, the child should lie on the side opposite the affected ear for 5 minutes after the drops are put in. If the child is older than 3 years, the pinna should be pulled up and back; if less than 3 years, pull it down and back.

47. a. The patient probably has impacted cerumen (earwax). This would explain the mild hearing loss and a sensation of fullness with intermittent ringing of the ears. Other assessments to make would include whether she has a history of ruptured tympanic membranes, auditory canal surgery, or myringotomy tubes, as these would contraindicate an ear irrigation and the use of earwax softeners.

    b. Initial nursing interventions would include removal by using mineral oil or an earwax softener preparation, followed by irrigation with a bulb syringe.